"Highly recommended for the novice user to get started on the right path, as well as [for] long-time aromatherapists. There's something for everyone in this book!"

—Sylla Sheppard-Hanger, LMT, founder and director of the
Atlantic Institute of Aromatherapy

"Beautifully designed and put together, you will refer to this book again and again."

—Dr. Steven Farmer, best-selling author of *Earth Magic*, *Animal Spirit Guides* and *Healing Ancestral Karma*

"I highly recommend to anyone that has an interest in aromatherapy and exploring the energetic and vibrational aspects of essential oils that they add this book to their aromatic library."

—Kelly Holland Azzaro, RA, CCAP, CBFP, LMT, registered aromatherapist, aromatherapy educator and past president of the National Association for Holistic Aromatherapy

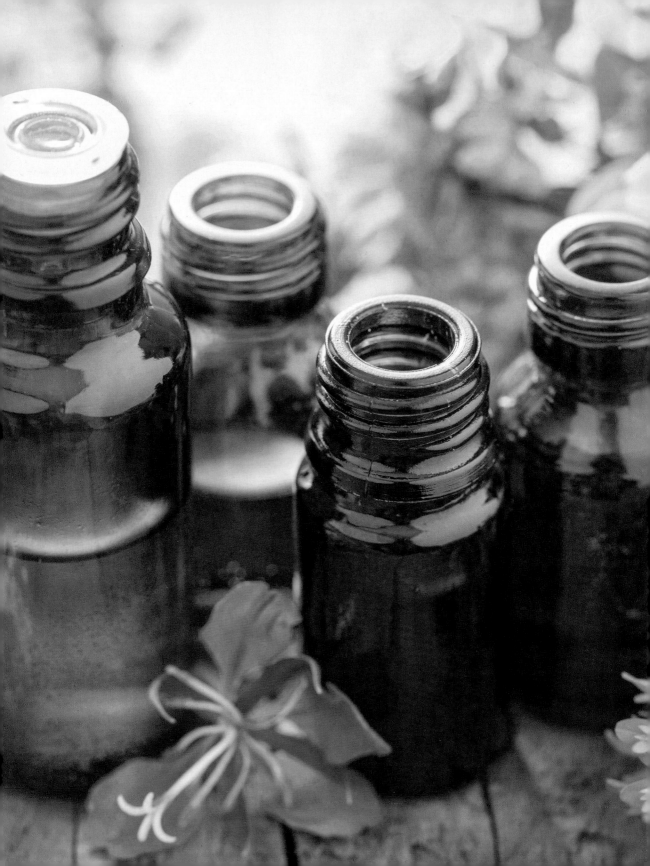

The Best
Natural Cures
Using Essential Oils

100 Remedies for Colds, Anxiety, Better Sleep and More

KG Stiles
BA, CBT, CBP, LMT
Aromatherapist to the Stars

PAGE STREET
PUBLISHING CO.

PAGE STREET
PUBLISHING CO.

First published in 2021 by
Page Street Publishing Co.
27 Congress Street, Suite 105
Salem, MA 01970
www.pagestreetpublishing.com

Distributed by Macmillan, sales in Canada by The Canadian Manda Group.

25 24 23 22 21   1 2 3 4 5

ISBN-13: 978-1-64567-318-7
ISBN-10: 1-64567-318-9

Library of Congress Control Number: 2020948786

Cover and book design by Page Street Publishing Co.

Photography Research by KG Stiles
Photos from Shutterstock on pages 2, 5, 7, 15, 17, 19, 22, 26, 27, 31, 33, 34, 36, 41, 45, 46, 50, 53, 54, 57, 61, 65, 66, 75, 76, 83, 89, 90, 95, 97, 99, 102, 106, 109, 111, 114, 117, 118, 122, 127, 135 and 139
Photos from iStock on pages 38, 45 (bottom right) and 70

Printed and bound in China

Page Street Publishing protects our planet by donating to nonprofits like The Trustees, which focuses on local land conservation.

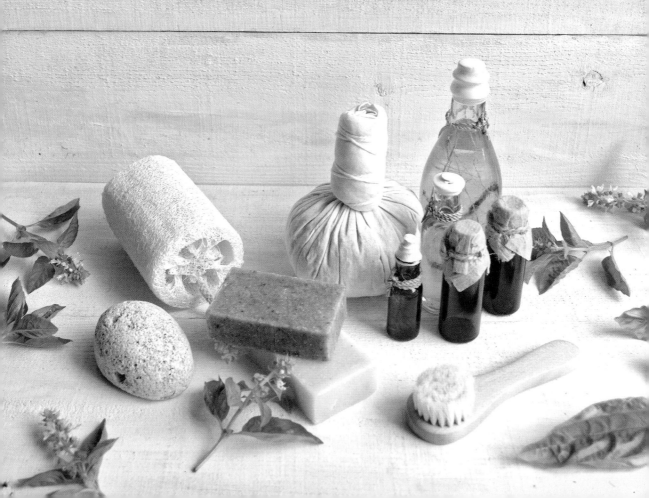

For my readers and fans.
You made all the years of incessant writing
and the piles of rejection letters
all worthwhile. Thank you!

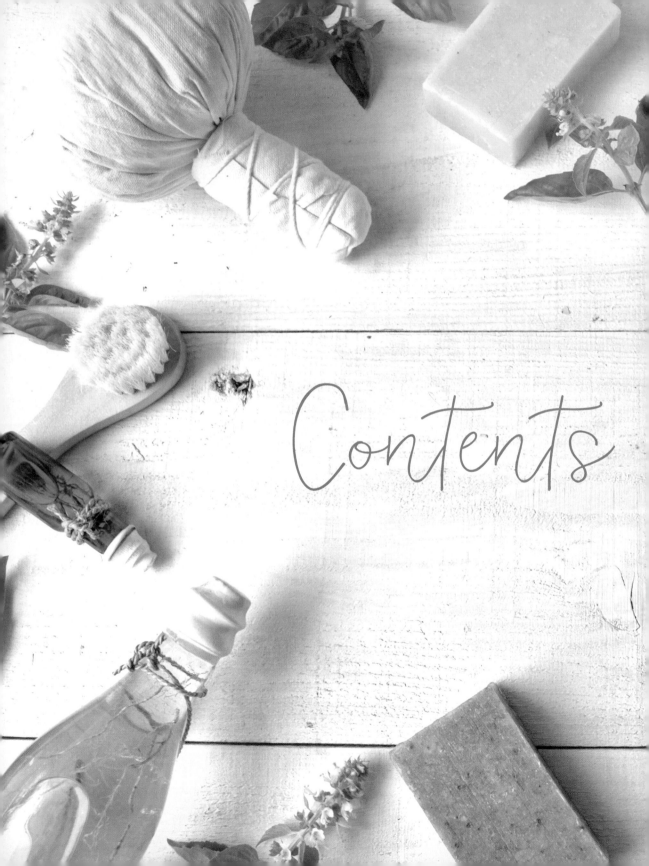

Contents

Introduction

My perspective, as a veteran in the metaphysical healing movement, is that everyone is on a healing journey during their lifetime. There's always some challenge that needs a solution. This is very apparent at the collective level where the repetition of patterns of war and strife are prevalent. Perhaps now at this seemingly critical moment in human history in which we've created such a multiplicity of challenges at the world level including global warming, overpopulation, massive poverty, rampant disease, world starvation and species extinction, there is an opportunity for a mass paradigm shift, a transformation in our way of thinking and behaving in which we move from competition to cooperation.

I believe we can look to nature for solutions to our individual and global challenges. Nature and natural life have been adapting to change and evolving for hundreds of thousands of years. If you observe nature you can see that she works holistically and in cooperation through cycles of time to sustain herself. Historically, when things get out of balance, there is massive die-off of species, and natural habitats shift to bring balance once again. I believe we are in one of those major points on planet Earth.

From the metaphysical perspective, everything is working perfectly to bring balance into the crisis point we are faced with on planet Earth. It's attuning to and aligning with natural forces to support them in this natural process of evolution that will help restore balance.

Transformation and healing are always available. It's our willingness to align with natural forces that guides us to see the opportunities available in our own personal life and for planetary evolution. Humans can be the stewards that allow this evolution to take place.

Essential oils can help with this process of transformation and change. On an individual level, when used properly, essential oils can act like trusted allies and friends to help you shift and handle any challenges you may be faced with—whether they be physical, mental, emotional or spiritual—in order to become more integrated and whole.

As a metaphysician and holistic healing practitioner, I've explored using many forms of transformation and healing. Over time I've come to focus solely on working with my clients at the metaphysical and energetic level. Your emotion is literally energy in motion. Resistance to feeling the energy expressed as your emotions creates stress in your body, and physical tension builds. Resistance and the suppression of emotions is at the core of most illness and disease. When you release the blocked patterns of emotional resistance, the natural process of transformation that's always available can occur to bring you back into balance, and healing occurs naturally.

Young children express the inner joy that comes with the experience of being alive. Children are naturally inquisitive and creative. Before age four, the majority of children test at genius level, and by age ten they test at average intelligence. The conditioning and indoctrination children experience results in suppression of their natural talents and abilities.

As I began exploring metaphysical healing, I was introduced to the transformational healing arts at Findhorn, a spiritual community in northern Scotland. Findhorn is one of the largest intentional communities in the world and a working eco-village that was created to inspire and encourage transformation in human consciousness. Findhorn is renowned for growing huge vegetables, produced in cooperation with nature spirits.

While at Findhorn, my communication with the Devic kingdom opened fully. It was like coming home to myself. After Findhorn, I relocated to San Diego, California, a mecca for evolving consciousness and learning about and practicing the healing arts. My own personal healing journey continued as I explored a wide variety of cutting-edge healing modalities. Having a direct personal experience of whatever I taught or used in my practice was essential for me. The same has been true with using essential oils.

Having so many of my own health challenges to heal has been a blessing in that I know firsthand what my client must face and overcome. Though each client is an individual and has their own personal experience, there are similar patterns that surface and must be exposed and released so that natural healing may occur.

Much of the healing journey is about forgiving and releasing the past. We make decisions often in early childhood about what things mean and get locked into perspectives, attitudes and beliefs about ourselves and life that can undermine our best attempts at creating a happy life for ourselves. We develop a storyline for our life. When we're affected by these patterns of thinking and behaving, we generate the same chemicals that create the same emotional set points. These emotional set points can hardwire us into feeling depressed or frustrated and angry most of the time. Emotional patterns can become chronic.

It's very simple to release these set points, though it can take time to fully cleanse your cup, so to speak, and to experience a paradigm shift and a new way of life for yourself. I'll cover more of this when I speak about the different oils and how they can specifically help you. You'll understand how to use essential oils to help you holistically at all levels of being: body, mind, spirit and emotions.

I'll share some of my own direct personal experiences about how I've used the oils with myself and my clients with outstanding results. I will also pepper in a few of my other preferred methods that will allow you to align with the transformation and healing that is always available to you.

Thanks for joining me for a glimpse into the world of essential oils.

KGStiles

Background Information
on Essential Oils

Essential oils are the concentrated volatile or ethereal oils extracted from a single botanical plant source. The part of the plant that yields the maximum amount of volatile oil is what's used in the extraction process, for example flowers, leaves, stems, bark, seeds or roots of shrubs, bushes, herbs and trees.

When the substance of scent is still in the plant, it is called an essence. After distillation from the plant part, the volatile aromatic compound is referred to as an essential oil.

These subtle, highly aromatic plant extracts are found in the specialized cells or glands of plants. Through millennia, these plant excretions have evolved as protection for a plant from predators and to attract pollinators. Surprisingly, aromatic compounds are not found in all plants. Why this is so remains a mystery.

Pure essential oils are most often extracted by steam distillation. Other methods of extraction include cold pressing and expression, solvent extraction, absolute oil extraction and resin tapping. Essential oils are used in manufacturing perfumes, cosmetics, soaps, pharmaceuticals, incense and household cleaning products, as well as to flavor food and drink.

Essential oils have a long history of use as medicinals. Their wide range of use includes treatments for beauty and skincare, cold and flu prevention and treatment, as well as natural remedies to treat a variety of health issues from respiratory conditions to digestive complaints, insomnia and even cancer, and also to aid in weight loss. Many of the reports are anecdotal in nature, though more and more evidence-based research is being done to corroborate their use. Some medical centers are incorporating essential oils as a part of an integrative health care system.

As the specific compounds and properties of essential oils are studied, there is greater understanding about why certain essential oils have particular actions and effects as natural health remedies.

What Is Aromatherapy?

During the early twentieth century, a French chemist by the name of René-Maurice Gattefossé began researching the medicinal properties of essential oils. It is Gattefossé who is credited with having coined the term "aromatherapy."

The story of Gattefossé accidentally burning his arm very badly while conducting an experiment in a perfumery plant is well known. There are different versions about how Gattefossé on "reflex" plunged his arm into a large vat of lavender. Whether he knew it was lavender or thought it was water, the story goes that Gattefossé experienced rapid healing of his burns with very little scarring of tissue.

In his article "Gattefossé's Burn," aromatherapist Robert Tisserand recounts the actual story that Gattefossé reports himself of the incident in his 1937 book, *Aromathérapie*. According to Tisserand, Gattefossé tells how he was covered with burning substances in a laboratory explosion that he "extinguished by rolling on a grassy lawn." Gattefossé tells how he rinsed both of his badly burned hands with lavender oil, which stopped "the gasification of the tissue" that had started. Gas gangrene is a serious and often fatal infection with a 20 to 25 percent mortality rate. Gattefossé further reported that he sweated profusely after the treatment with lavender essence and that his hands showed signs of healing by the very next day.

As essential oils are highly aromatic, many of their benefits are obtained simply through inhalation. Our sense of smell is closely linked to memory, mood and emotion. It is well known that aroma reaches and influences our deepest primitive instincts. When essential oils are diffused and inhaled, aromatherapy not only delivers the calming benefits of fragrance, but also delivers many health benefits unique to essential oils.

The use of plants and herbs is the oldest form of healing disease and pain, and the medicinal effects of plants have been recorded in the oldest writings in history, myth and folklore. Records found in ancient Egyptian hieroglyphics and Chinese manuscripts show that priests and physicians were using plant aromatics thousands of years before the birth of Christ to heal the sick and infirm.

In ancient times, certain plant balms and fragrances like frankincense and myrrh were considered more valuable than gold. There are numerous references to plant substances in the Bible. Now, with the advent of modern scientific research, we are beginning to investigate the incredible healing potential found in essential oils.

Virtually everything used today in modern drugs can be traced back to a botanical extract. Hippocrates, the father of modern medicine, taught that following traditional healing wisdom and common sense passed down to us for thousands of years in the use of botanical medicines is the best way to health and healing. He recommended a scented bath and daily massage.

Brief History of Aromatherapy

The use of aromatic plants has been around since Neolithic times. It is thought that "smudging" was the earliest form of aromatic treatment, and it is very likely that shamans and priests were the first aromatherapists and perfumers. Medicinal plants have been found inside graves dating back eighty thousand years; however, the use of pure essential oils as we know them today has only been available since the creation of distillation.

The earliest devices for distilling oils were found in the ancient Indus Valley dating to 3000 BC, where terra cotta distillation devices and perfume containers were discovered. Since that time, plant aromatics have been used in every aspect of Indian culture, including beauty treatments, perfuming, medicinal practices, cleansing and ritual bathing and religious ceremonies. Traditionally, Indian tantric practices have been used to anoint the body with oils to seduce and arouse the passions. The Vedas, some of the most ancient sacred texts known, contained formulas for plant aromatics. The Rig Veda contained instructions for how to use over 700 aromatic plants, including spikenard, myrrh, sandalwood, ginger, cinnamon and coriander. Humans were seen as part of nature, and the

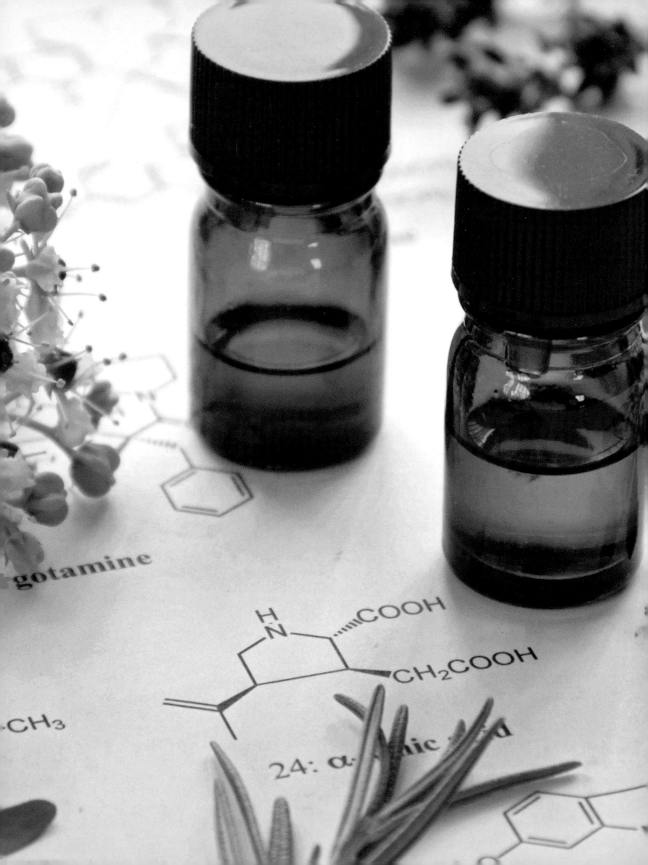

gotamine

H
N
‴COOH

CH₂COOH

·CH₃

24: α-ᵢₙᵢc ᵢd

preparation of plant medicinals was considered a sacred art and practice. Ayurvedic medicine is one of the oldest forms of medicine practiced continuously since ancient times.

In 1868, the first synthetic fragrance oils were produced. These synthetic fragrances were considered unsuitable for medicinal use. Chemists began to isolate the active ingredients within aromatic plants and manufacture them synthetically. Manufactured chemical drugs acted more powerfully and were cheaper to produce. As science became more sophisticated, herbs and essential oils were replaced by synthetic drugs.

By the 1900s, medical doctors became accustomed to using synthetic chemicals, and aromatic oils almost completely disappeared in the Western world.

In the mid-twentieth century, there was a renewed interest in essential oils, and they were used extensively as flavoring, perfumes, cosmetics and household cleaning supplies. Essential oils were commonly used in medicine and in a wide range of pharmaceutical products to mask the strong odor of the chemicals.

In 1964, French ex-army surgeon Jean Valnet published *The Practice of Aromatherapy,* which was written for laypeople as well as medical professionals. Valnet had used essential oils for treating wounded soldiers and found them to be highly effective for treating wounds and burns.

During this same time, Madame Maury, an Austrian-born biochemist who was influenced by Valnet's research, wrote *The Secret of Life and Youth,* a self-help, holistic approach to beauty using aromatherapy.

Robert Tisserand's book, *The Art of Aromatherapy,* published in England in 1977, was the first book to combine medical and esoteric approaches to aromatherapy.

Since then, there has continued to be a renewed interest in aromatic oils, and aromatherapy is enjoying increased popular interest and use by the general public.

Aromatherapy Terms

Adulterant: A substance that was not originally present in the oil at the time of distillation that is added to an essential oil. An adulterant can be artificial or natural.

Aromatherapy Massage: A hands-on therapy in which essential oils are applied to the body for emotional and physical benefits.

Carrier Oil: Vegetable or nut oils such as light coconut oil, jojoba, sweet almond and grapeseed, used to dilute essential oils.

Cold-Press Extraction or Expression: The cold-pressed method of extraction is one of the best methods for extracting essential oils as there is very little heat applied with this process. Cold pressing or expression applies a mechanical method of extraction in which no external heat is needed for the process. With cold pressing, essential oils are obtained by mechanically pressing the fruit peel. The downside of essential oils produced by cold pressing is that they usually have a very short shelf life. Citrus oils like grapefruit, lemon and orange are obtained by cold-press extraction.

Diffuser: A device that disperses essential oils into an area. The three basic types are clay, candle and electric.

Dilute: Adding a small amount of essential oil to a larger amount of base oil to make it safe for use on the skin.

Distillation: A method used to extract essential oil from the plant. Steam distillation is the most common form of distillation.

Essential Oil: A highly aromatic substance found in specialized cells of certain plants. Technically, when this substance is in the plant, it is called an "essence." After distillation of a single type of plant, the aromatic substance is referred to as an essential oil.

Expression: See Cold-Press Extraction or Expression.

Extraction Method: The method by which essential oils are separated from the plant. Common extraction methods include steam distillation, expression and solvent extraction.

Fixative: A fixative is a plant or animal substance of low volatility that serves to draw together and hold the fragrances of other materials. It may be in the form of a liquid, such as an essential oil or fragrance, that will slow the evaporation process and preserve the aromatic scent of the blend, or it may be in the form of a botanical that will absorb and hold the various aromas. Using a fixative will create a more distinct and longer-lasting product. Orris root, amyris, calamus root, angelica root and vetiver root are a few commonly used fixatives.

Food Grade: Considered safe for use in food by the Food and Drug Administration (FDA).

Fragrance: Aroma products labeled as fragrances are not the same as essential oils. Fragrances are derived by synthetic means, while essential oils are completely natural.

GC/MS (Gas Chromatograph/Mass Spectrometer): A device used by analytic chemists to determine the precise makeup of a given substance. It is used in aromatherapy to determine the precise chemical constituents of an essential oil and whether the oil is pure or adulterated with synthetic chemicals or other products.

Herbal Infused Oils: Oils made through the extraction of volatile oils of a plant, which are obtained by soaking the plant in a carrier oil for approximately two weeks and then straining off the oils from the plant material. The resulting oil is infused with the plant's aromatic characteristic actions and effects and used therapeutically.

Herbal Medicine (Herbalism): Pertaining to natural botanicals and living plants in various forms or preparations. They are valued for their therapeutic benefits and sold as dietary supplements.

Hydrosol: The name for the water left after steam or water distillation of an essential oil. It is mainly water with only a very small amount of water-soluble plant constituents.

Infused Oil: These are oils that carry the medicinal properties of certain herbs. Carrier oil is infused with the medicinal herb, the plant is strained off and the remaining oil can be used directly on the skin.

Insoluble: Unable to be dissolved in a liquid such as water.

Liniment: Extract of a plant added to either alcohol or vinegar and applied topically for therapeutic benefits.

Neat: An undiluted essential oil.

Notes: As in *top*, *middle* and *base* notes. A type of classification system based on aroma to identify certain oils. Generally, essential oils from citrus peels are top notes; essential oils from flowers, leaves and stems are middle notes; and essential oils from roots are base notes.

Olfactory: Relating to, or connected with, the sense of smell.

Orifice Reducer: A device used to reduce the size of the opening of a bottle, making dispensing the essential oil easier and more accurate.

Patch Test: A test to assess for sensitivity to an oil. To patch test an essential oil you haven't used before, add one drop of essential oil to a half teaspoon of vegetable carrier oil. Apply to the back of a knee or inside of an arm, and then cover with a bandage and leave it on for twenty-four hours. If any redness, swelling or itching occurs, don't use the oil.

Phytochemicals: Chemical compounds or constituents that are formed in the plant's normal metabolic processes. Often referred to as "secondary metabolites," there are many classes of plant distillates. When isolated from the plant, these chemicals are considered pharmaceutical drugs.

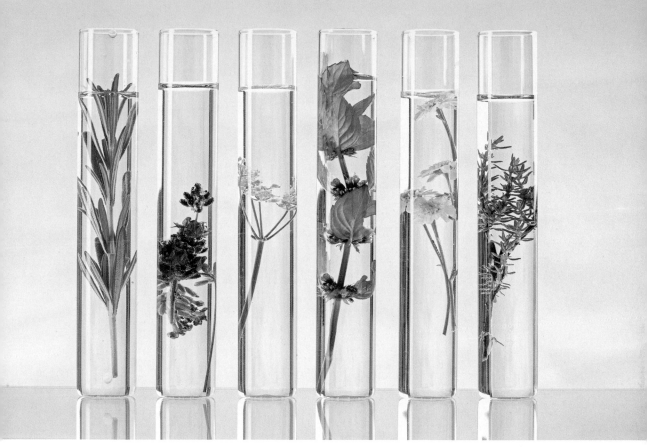

Herbal infused oils carry the plant's aromatic characteristics.

Phytomedicinals: Medical substances that originate from plants.

Poultice: Therapeutic topical application of plant material or plant extract, usually wrapped in a fine woven cloth for therapeutic benefits.

Sebum: The oily substance produced by the sebaceous glands, which function to lubricate the skin and seal moisture into the cells. The level of sebum production determines whether your skin is normal, dry or oily.

Single Note: An essential oil from a single botanical source without any other ingredients.

Soluble: Able to dissolve in a liquid such as water.

Synergistic: A characteristic effect in which the sum total is more effective than the individual parts.

Synthetic: An imitation or artificial reproduction of a naturally occurring substance.

Viscosity: Relates to the thickness or thinness of an essential oil.

Volatile: Describes how quickly a substance disperses (evaporates) into the air. In aromatherapy, top note essential oils may be referred to as "highly volatile," meaning that they disperse quickly out of the bottle and into the air.

Volatilization: The rate of evaporation or oxidation of an essential oil.

CHAPTER 2

How Aromatherapy Works

As more and more research is being done that shows the effectiveness of using essential oils as an alternative health care system, there is a growing demand by the public for information.

At the same time, more and more people are taking responsibility for their health, which is fueling a growing revolution in the "Do-It-Yourself" movement. The practice of aromatherapy truly lends itself to this new holistic health culture, where we want to freely choose the health care systems we use, spawning a new vision of health care in our future.

With new scientific studies providing evidence of the benefits of using essential oils, there is an increasing demand from people that hospitals and medical centers offer safe alternatives to allopathic drugs, which can produce harmful side effects. As a result, hospitals are beginning to offer integrative health care to patients.

Nurses and staff are receiving training and certification in the effective and safe use of essential oils as a comfort care measure for their patients and are reporting outstanding results.

Essential oils are super-concentrated plant extracts (one drop is equal to 3 to 4 cups [121 to 161 g] of raw plant matter). This super concentration means that only a single drop or two of an essential oil is needed for achieving therapeutic benefits, making the use of essential oils extremely cost-effective. In today's world of rising health costs, this is a significant benefit to using essential oils because a little goes a long way.

Research has shown that most of the therapeutic benefits from essential oils can be experienced simply by inhaling them. This makes the use of essential oils extremely efficient.

In the use of essential oils, the meeting of the elements of heat, light, air and moisture activates the release of their scent. Interestingly, scent bypasses your logical brain, which is not at all involved in your process of smell. You actually "feel" the scent of an essential oil.

Research has also shown that essential oils act as powerful chemicals to trigger the limbic part of your brain that controls emotions, memory and mood.

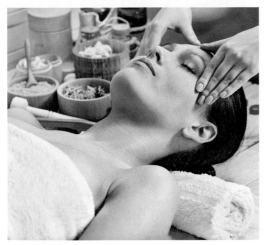

Inhalation of essential oils from an aromatherapy massage can effect an immediate relaxation response.

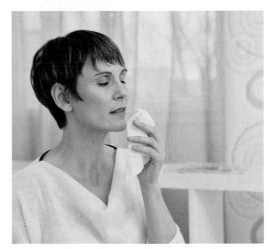

A woman inhales the scent of an essential oil.

Upon inhaling the scent of an essential oil, the vapors enter through your nose and immediately stimulate your olfactory nerve. The olfactory nerve instantaneously signals your limbic system (control center for emotions), the amygdala and hippocampus (control centers for memory, learning and emotions), which then respond by releasing chemicals such as serotonin that produce a calming effect (refer to chart "The Electrochemical Effects of Aromatherapy" [page 23]).

At the same time, your limbic system sends a signal to your cortex (control center for intellectual processes) and to your hypothalamus gland, located at the base of your brain. Also known as the reptilian or old brain, the hypothalamus regulates many body functions including appetite, thirst, temperature, sleep and mood.

Regulating the conversation between your nervous and hormonal systems, the hypothalamus sends a signal to your pituitary gland, the master controller of your entire endocrine system. This cascade of neuro-chemical signals and responses ends at your adrenal glands, which control your fight or flight response, aggression and sexual response.

Essential oils also work through your blood vascular system, which delivers them to all of your organs and systems. The vapors entering through your nose go immediately into your lungs where they enter your bloodstream and are delivered to your heart, as well as all of your other organs and tissues. The oils then circulate back to your lungs where they are expelled.

The best delivery method to benefit the skin, muscles, soft tissues and joints is through skin application using a vegetable carrier oil. As essential oils are extremely concentrated and may cause skin irritation if applied neat to the skin, they should always be diluted for safe skin application.

CHAPTER 3

How to Use
Essential Oils

Therapeutic Use of Essential Oils: Delivery Methods for Best Results

Pure essential oils have a wide range of therapeutic uses and benefits. The method applied can affect the results. Your choice of delivery method often depends upon your intended goal.

There are three ways to use essential oils: internally, externally and environmentally. Please refer to the chart diagram "Aromatherapy Delivery Pathways" (page 21) illustrating the three ways of using essential oils, as well as their pathways of distribution and the organs and systems being affected.

Direct Inhalation Method

This is one of the quickest, easiest, least expensive and most effective ways to use and benefit from essential oils.

How close together can you use an essential oil or blend? Generally you can use essential oils within half an hour or so of each other; it depends on an individual's absorption and response rate. Increasing your heart rate just prior to direct inhalation will enhance the absorption rate of the oils.

For optimal results, follow these guidelines

Dispense 1 to 3 drops of essential oil onto a cotton ball, smell strip, tissue or dram vial of Celtic salts. Close your eyes and inhale as you gently and slowly introduce the oil's aromatic vapors into your system. Take four slow, full deep breaths for up to 10 to 30 seconds to begin. Inhale for a slow count of 1-2-3-4 and exhale for a slow count of 1-2-3-4.

Breathe in slowly and pause briefly on your inhaled breath. Then slowly exhale, letting go of any tension. Repeat this slow, rhythmic breathing pattern for four cycles of breathing. If you feel lightheaded or dizzy at any time, allow yourself to rest before continuing. After direct inhalation, allow yourself to relax for a moment into a feeling of well-being.

The aromatic vapors of the essential oils work through both your hormonal and circulatory systems to produce their effects. Please refer to the chart diagram for "The Electrochemical Effects of Aromatherapy" (page 23) and the "How Aromatherapy Works" chapter (page 18) to find out more.

Aromatherapy Delivery Pathways

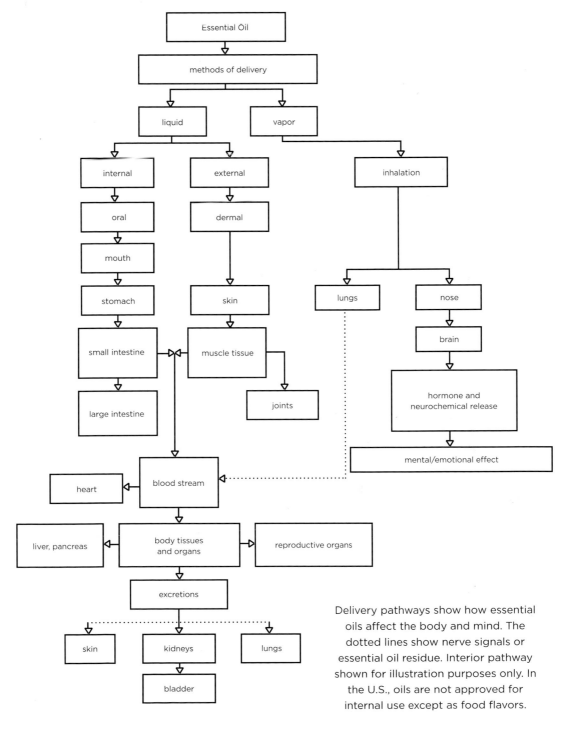

Delivery pathways show how essential oils affect the body and mind. The dotted lines show nerve signals or essential oil residue. Interior pathway shown for illustration purposes only. In the U.S., oils are not approved for internal use except as food flavors.

Cold-Air Diffusion

For cold-air diffusion, drops of essential oil are dispensed onto a cotton or wool pad in the diffuser compartment. A small fan then blows cool air through the oils, lifting them into the air for dispersal into the environment. This is a cost-effective way for diffusing your oils into the atmosphere of a room. Cold-air diffusion has the benefits of micro diffusion and is especially good for scenting a room without the cleanup time required with a nebulizing diffuser, especially when using thicker oils.

Environmental Fragrance

Research has shown that cold-air diffusing certain oils into the environment may:

- Reduce bacteria, fungus, mold and unpleasant odor.
- Relax and relieve tension, as well as clear the mind.
- Assist with weight management.
- Improve concentration, alertness and mental clarity.

Start by diffusing your essential oils for fifteen to thirty minutes per day. As you become accustomed to the oils and recognize their effects, you may increase your time of exposure to them.

Ultrasonic Micro Diffusion

Micro diffusion uses a nebulizing type of diffuser that breaks down essential oils into millions of micro particles. This type of diffusion disperses oils without the heating that can render oils less therapeutically beneficial.

In illness, you may consider inhaling the oil's vapors near the "mouth" of the nebulizer. A short session of breathing in the oils for four to five minutes should be sufficient; repeat every few hours.

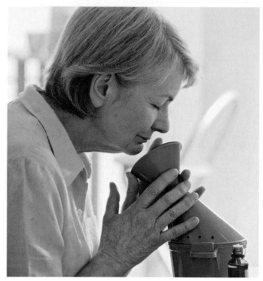

A woman inhales aromatic vapors from a wide-mouthed (electric) diffuser.

Facial Steam

For your personal skincare, a facial steam with select essential oils plays a key role in any deep cleansing and healing skincare routine. A facial steam uses the trapped vapors from hot water to cleanse the skin. It adds moisture to the skin and loosens toxins from the skin's pores. A facial steam is also very therapeutic for all of your five senses, as well as for relaxing your body and mind.

Extraordinarily easy to do, a facial steam takes very little time to perform. Once a month for five to fifteen minutes is all that's required to get excellent results.

All you need for an at-home facial steam is a small ceramic or stainless steel bowl to which you add hot water (up to 102°F [39°C]), adding your essential oils in a suitable carrier like cream or honey. With a towel draped over your head and eyes closed, you will lean over the bowl of steaming water face forward. The towel will catch the steam from the hot water so that it penetrates the facial skin.

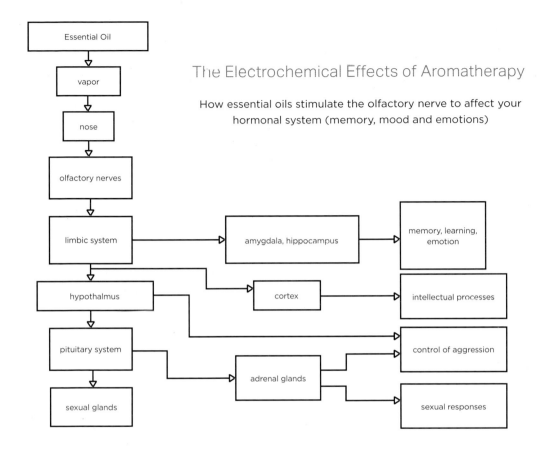

The Electrochemical Effects of Aromatherapy

How essential oils stimulate the olfactory nerve to affect your hormonal system (memory, mood and emotions)

The amount of time you take to do your facial steam treatment is specific to you and depends upon your comfort level with the steam, but generally takes between five to fifteen minutes.

You can also use your essential oils in facial steaming machines that are commonly used at spas, which you can also purchase for at-home use.

Before performing a facial steam you will usually want to cleanse your face to remove any excess oil, dirt or makeup, which can clog pores, in order to make the most of your facial steam experience.

Once you've completed your facial, towel dry your skin and wipe your face with a facial toner to remove any sweat and cool down the skin. (Refer to the Spa and Beauty Treatments section of this book on page 104 for guidelines on making your own facial toner with essential oils.)

PLEASE NOTE: Essential oils are not water soluble. You must use a dispersant when adding them to a facial steam. Hot water may cause essential oils to penetrate your system more quickly or cause irritation to sensitive or damaged skin, like blemishes, sores or rashes.

Respiratory Steam

Although facial steams are often performed primarily for cosmetic reasons, they can also offer extraordinary medicinal benefits for your respiratory system. You can use steam to effectively soothe cold or flu symptoms like sore throats, nasal congestion and other respiratory symptoms.

CAUTION: If you have serious respiratory issues like asthma, it is recommended that you consult with a health professional or doctor before using a steam that contains any aromatic herbs or essential oils to ensure they won't cause irritation or other breathing complications.

Dilution Guide

The first step in making aromatherapy products is to understand the concept of dilution.

The principle idea is to dilute essential oils for safe skin application. Remember, each drop of pure essential oil is very concentrated. One drop of pure essential oil is equivalent to about 1 to 4 cups (26 to 104 g) of dried plant matter. As pure essential oils are very concentrated, some essential oils can cause skin irritation if used undiluted. Additionally, some people may have sensitivity to certain chemical properties in an essential oil. When first using an essential oil never used before, it is advised to do a simple skin test.

See Chapter 7 (page 52) for "Aromatherapy Formulas."

Safe Skin Application

How much essential oil should you put into your carrier for safe skin application?

Generally, effective blends for adults are made using a dilution ratio of 1, 2 or 3 percent of essential oil to carrier. Perfume oils usually have a higher dilution ratio of 5 to 10 percent.

1% dilution: 5–6 drops essential oil per 1 ounce (30 ml) carrier oil

Use for children under age twelve, seniors over sixty-five, pregnant women and people with long-term illnesses or immune system disorders. A 1 percent dilution is a good place to start with individuals who are generally sensitive to aromas, chemicals or other environmental pollutants.

2% dilution: 10–12 drops essential oil per 1 ounce (30 ml) carrier oil

Use for general health and skincare, natural perfumes, bath products and for your everyday blends.

3% dilution: 15–18 drops essential oil per 1 ounce (30 ml) carrier oil

Use for specific application blends and acute health conditions such as cold, flu or pain relief and for sports blends.

5% dilution: 28–30 drops essential oil per 1 ounce (30 ml) carrier oil

Use for sports massage blends, natural perfumes and short-term treatment for specific, acute health conditions.

10% dilution: 58–60 drops essential oil per 1 ounce (30 ml) carrier oil

Very expensive essential oils like rose, helichrysum and neroli pure essential oils are often made available in a 10 percent dilution of carrier oil. Essential oil blends for natural colognes, perfumes and other specific applications may also be found in 10 percent dilutions. If you're using a 10 percent dilution of any of the pure essential oils, add them directly to your bottle of carrier oil before application instead of adding them to a synergy blend.

When making larger quantities of blends of 3 ounces (90 ml) or more, you can try using less essential oil than recommended above. You may find that doubling amounts of essential oils is not necessary for effectiveness when making larger quantities of blended oils.

Face Carrier Oils

Essential oils are diluted in suitable carriers like oils, lotions, creams, salts and clays to make your products. Generally, whatever will absorb an essential oil and is safe for skin application can be used as a carrier to make your health and beauty treatments.

Water is not an acceptable carrier for essential oil that is being applied directly to the skin, since oil and water do not mix. For general safe use on the skin, it is always best to dilute your essential oil in an oil-based carrier or other suitable carrier; it should be one that will absorb and carry your essential oil.

A 5-milliliter, euro-dropper bottle contains approximately 100 drops of liquid. A 1 percent dilution of essential oil would be 1 drop to 99 drops of carrier oil. Please refer to the "Safety and Dilution Guide" on page 140.

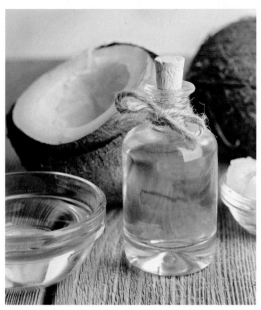

Coconut oil is closest in molecular structure to skin's own natural sebum.

Choose oils that are skin nourishing and healing like pure fractionated coconut oil or jojoba. Both of these oils act as excellent carriers of essential oil. Coconut oil has the added benefit of being fully metabolized by the body, helping it to be absorbed through the fatty tissues beneath the skin and into the blood stream. Diluting your essential oil in a carrier also helps you avoid any possible skin irritation.

Fractionated Coconut Oil

(Cocos nucifera)

I highly recommend using this oil, also called light coconut oil, as the ideal carrier for most of your topical essential oil body and face applications.

Light coconut oil is one of the most effective natural body moisturizers available. I've used light coconut oil in all my personal skincare products for many years and absolutely love the results I experience for myself and my customers. It makes a great base for sensitive skincare products, and its "light" texture makes it suitable for all skin types, especially for dry, itchy, inflamed or sensitive skin. Excellent for nail and cuticle treatments, use light coconut oil as a base for essential oils, on your skin as a moisturizer, after exposure to the sun and at night before bed to nourish your skin. Its cooling and moisturizing action serve to protect your skin while helping it retain moisture.

Light coconut oil's softening and lubricating effects on the skin are excellent for treating conditions that a "totally natural" carrier oil might actually exacerbate. For instance, when using essential oils to treat damaged skin, a totally natural carrier oil could potentially introduce molds, bacteria or fungi to the skin, making the condition worse, whereas using a refined and sterilized carrier oil like light coconut oil can actually prevent further problems and promote beneficial results.

Unique Qualities of Fractionated Coconut Oil

1. Coconut oil is fully metabolized by the body and, unlike most oils, is not absorbed into the fat cell tissues of the body. This makes it an ideal carrier for essential oils to move through the fat cells beneath the dermis and into the blood vessels serving the muscles and soft tissues.

2. Light coconut oil remains liquid at room temperature. You may be familiar with the pure, whole coconut oil, which solidifies at room temperature, but may not have yet experienced light fractionated coconut oil, which uses a simple, non-chemical physical process to separate the smaller fatty acid triglycerides from the whole coconut oil to produce fractionated coconut oil.

3. Along with jojoba oil, light coconut oil shares the distinction of being closest in molecular structure to your skin's own natural sebum, making it more readily absorbed into your skin and ideal for use in natural skincare and for massage therapy.

4. Its light consistency will not clog skin pores, making it suitable to use on dry, oily, sensitive or problem skin.

5. Light coconut oil has such a light consistency that it easily washes out of most fabrics, table linens, sheets and towels, making it ideal for massage therapy.

6. Due to its molecular structure, light coconut oil is not subject to oxidation. This means that it has an almost infinite shelf life with almost no possibility of going rancid.

7. Its anti-fungal properties make light coconut oil especially suitable for use in your fungicidal essential oil blends—for example, athlete's foot treatment.

8. Light or fractionated coconut oil is produced by heat, rather than cold pressing, which deodorizes the oil. Being odorless, light coconut oil makes an ideal carrier for aromatic oils. You can use it for making perfume oils and 10 percent dilutions of more expensive pure essential oils. This allows you to enjoy the pure scent of the oil without interference from the scent of your carrier oil.

9. Light coconut oil adds a silky, smooth, light quality to other more expensive carrier oils like jojoba.

10. Its consistency is so light you can use it in a spray bottle for misting on skin applications, and it won't clog your atomizer pump.

Of course when you prefer using a natural oil, there are some excellent choices for you.

Organic Jojoba Oil

(Simmondsia californica)

Jojoba oil is more like a wax in its consistency and composition than an oil, and closely resembles your skin's own natural sebum. Because of its close resemblance, jojoba readily penetrates through your skin cell tissue and won't clog pores, making it an excellent choice for beauty and skincare treatments.

Unique Qualities of Jojoba Oil

1. Because of its compatibility with your skin tissue, jojoba oil is highly nourishing for all skin types.

2. Its anti-inflammatory properties have a soothing effect on irritated or inflamed skin cells and connective tissues.

3. Jojoba oil's regulating action makes it excellent for use in reconditioning skin, hair and scalp.

4. As a natural antioxidant, jojoba oil is one of the longest-lasting carrier oils, after light fractionated coconut oil.

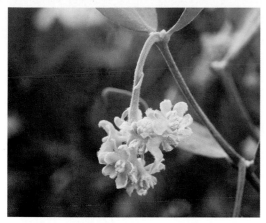

A natural antioxidant, jojoba oil is one of the longest-lasting carrier oils.

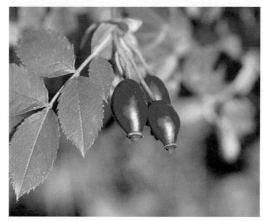

Avoid using rosehip oil with excessively oily skin types prone to acne outbreaks.

Rosehip Seed Oil

(Rosa rubiginosa)

High in gamma linolenic and other acids known to nourish and heal skin, rosehip seed oil has an excellent reputation for treating severe skin conditions like dry, cracked and aging skin, as well as treating traumatized skin issues like burns, ulcers, wounds and uneven or excessive pigmentation. You can add rosehip seed oil to your less expensive carrier oils to get all the benefits of rosehip oil without the higher cost.

CAUTION: Avoid using with excessively oily skin types prone to acne outbreaks.

Body Massage Carrier Oils

My top two carrier oils for body massage therapy are fractionated light coconut oil and jojoba for the same reasons that I recommend them for face massage.

Sweet Almond Oil

(Prunus amygdalus var. dulcis)

Rich in protein and other vitamins and minerals, sweet almond oil is suitable for all skin types and helpful for relieving dry, itchy skin, as well as for soothing inflammatory conditions like arthritis, fibromyalgia, injuries and burns. Sweet almond oil has been recommended as a remedy for treating dark circles and bags under your eyes.

Sesame Oil

(Sesamum indicum)

Skin-nourishing sesame oil is excellent for stimulating circulation and warming the body and internal organs. Sesame oil contains the antioxidant and anti-inflammatory compound sesamol that can promote heart health by preventing atherosclerotic lesions. A great conductor of electro-magnetic flow, sesame oil promotes balance and harmony of the mind and emotions. It is good for all skin types and useful for soothing a wide range of inflammatory conditions. Sesame is good for the skin both topically and internally. Sesame seeds contain anti-cancer compounds including phytic acid, magnesium and phytosterols.

Vitamin E Oil

(alpha-Tocopherol)

An antioxidant and natural preservative, vitamin E oil can be used to extend the life of your massage oils and prevent rancidity. Studies have shown immunity levels improve when vitamin E is consumed. Another important benefit of vitamin E is that it reduces cholesterol and the risk of developing cancer.

Wheat Germ Oil

(Triticum vulgare)

Another natural preservative for extending the life of your massage oils, wheat germ oil is an excellent source of minerals, protein, vitamin A, vitamin D, B vitamins, antioxidants and fatty acids. These nutrients are known to moisturize and heal dry, cracked and prematurely aging skin, as well as to help prevent scarring.

Bath

Hippocrates—considered one of the most influential figures in the history of medicine and referred to as the "Father of Western Medicine"—is credited as having said, "The way to health is to have an aromatic bath and scented massage every day." First and foremost, Hippocrates respected the healing forces of nature working within every living organism. Unlike his predecessors, Hippocrates believed that illness was a natural phenomenon that forces us to discover the imbalances occurring within our own life. His holistic approach to illness entailed a rigorous examination of his patients' daily habits and routines to understand what might be leading to an imbalanced health condition, manifesting as a disease.

Research shows that a warm bath is the most effective way to boost your serotonin levels and cleanse and detoxify your body and entire energy system.

Serotonin has been called the happiness hormone. It regulates your mood, appetite and sleep. Serotonin also improves your cognitive functions like memory and learning.

Healing baths and aromatic plants have been used since antiquity for ritual purification, cleansing and healing practices and to restore the human energy system—body, mind, spirit and emotions. As human beings, we are primarily made of water and have a natural affinity with water as a healing agent. Water represents your emotions. When your emotions flow, your energy stays in motion. The meridian energy system for cycling prana (or life force energy) becomes clogged when you resist and suppress feeling your emotions. Taking a warm water bath naturally frees your emotions.

Natural sea salts are frequently recommended for use as the carrier for essential oil in your healing baths. Salt has been prized for its healing properties since ancient times. During the Middle Ages, salt was at the heart of the spice trade industry, highly traded as a commodity and considered as priceless as gold. Sea salts are rich in minerals and charged with electrical healing properties that you can especially benefit from in a warm bath. Sea salts are inexpensive and readily available in your local health-food store in the bulk spice section.

Enjoying the daily holistic habit of a scented bath promotes regular restful sleep, increased energy and natural weight loss, as well as an enlivened sense of well-being and renewed passion for your life.

If you're someone who wants to live your genius and grow personally and professionally, as well as leave behind feelings of stress and over-exhaustion, I invite you to commit to a forty-day program of daily scented baths. This will allow you to reboot and rebalance your life and experience firsthand the dramatic changes that can occur. I've now taken a daily aromatic bath for more than four years, and I would not be where I am without it.

Radical self-care is critical if you are to thrive in today's fast-paced environment and create a work–life balance that allows you to live your best life. It has never been more important than now to take extraordinary care of yourself. Come back to yourself and enjoy being alive in the moment with a daily aromatherapy bath. Find out the exact essential oils recipe to use and instructions for your forty-day program for a daily aromatic bath in the "Spa and Beauty Treatments" section on page 104.

PLEASE NOTE: Essential oils are not water-soluble, and you must use a dispersant when adding them to a bath. The water may cause the oils to penetrate your system more quickly or cause irritation to sensitive or damaged skin (such as open wounds, blemishes, sores or rashes).

Compress

An essential oil compress can be applied directly to an area of the body, including an injury, wound or rash to:

1. Stem the flow of bleeding.
2. Relieve pain.
3. Speed recovery.
4. Promote healing.

Drops of essential oils are added to a bowl of hot or cold water and then absorbed in steril-ized material, like a cotton wash cloth or gauze. This is then applied with pressure to a part of the body to control bleeding or to supply heat, cold, moisture or therapeutic medicinal benefits in order to alleviate inflammation and pain or to reduce infection.

Compresses are excellent for topical application to ease pain from strained muscles, headaches, poison oak, menstrual cramps and more.

Poultice

A poultice is a soft, moist mass of material, typically made of absorbent plant material or flour, that is applied to an area of the body and kept in place with a cloth or bandage. Commonly used as a "drawing salve," a poultice is applied to wounds, cuts or injuries to increase circulation and relieve soreness, inflammation or infection. An essential oil poultice is usually made of heated water to which flour or bran with drops of essential oil has been added. The mixture is then spread on soft cloth and applied over the area requiring treatment.

A common treatment used on horses to relieve inflammation, a poultice can be used on any area of the body where you want to focus your treatment. Poultices can be applied as a precau-tionary measure to prevent injury after a hard workout. Effective for treating abscesses and wounds, use poultices where there is excessive discharge or build-up of pus needing to be drawn out.

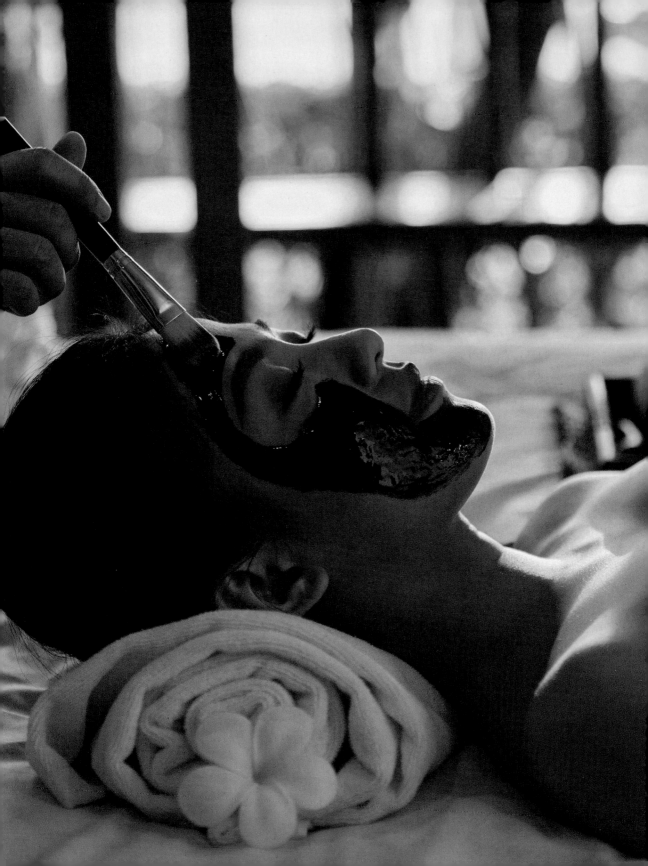

Masks and Wraps

Facial Masks

A facial mask treatment enlivens your skin cells and provides numerous other benefits. An essential oil facial mask covers your face or part of your face with a carrier like green or pink clay. Other carriers you can try include honey, cream, oats, avocado and egg whites. Your facial mask can take as little as 10–15 minutes, and the time is well worth the pleasure of caring for yourself and getting healthier skin.

Benefits

- Cleanses and detoxifies skin.
- Renews and nourishes skin cell tissue.
- Balances your skin's pH.
- Improves skin elasticity.
- Reduces fine lines and wrinkles.
- Imparts a radiant, youthful and healthy glow.

Body Wrap

Feel clean inside and out with an essential oil body wrap treatment. An aromatherapy body wrap involves the application of essential oils in a carrier like green or pink clay. Mud can also be used as a base to which you can add seaweed, water, aloe vera and salt. This is followed by wrapping the body or body part being treated with a sheet and then covering the area with blankets to create a warm, cocoon-like effect to activate and assist the cleansing, detoxification and healing process. Heat can also be applied to increase the natural detox of sweating. You can allow at least an hour and a half for a full body wrap experience, which includes time for a cleansing shower followed by a 10-minute period of resting afterward to get the most from your treatment.

For the best cleansing results for your skin and internal organs, it's best to do your body wrap in conjunction with a detoxing diet or whole body cleanse.

Benefits

- Cleanses, detoxifies and draws out impurities. Can help eliminate harmful toxins from your body and internal organs, as well as provide essential vitamins and minerals to your body's largest and most vulnerable organ, your skin.
- Nourishes the skin.
- Tightens and tones.
- Exfoliates and acts as an astringent, eliminating dead skin.
- Destroys harmful bacteria and fungus.
- Renews skin cell tissues.
- Increases circulation.
- Soothes, moisturizes and softens skin.
- Helps you absorb the beneficial qualities of essential oils.

Scrubs and Body Butters

Facial and Body Scrubs

Popularly known to promote a healthy, beautiful and youthful appearance, scrubs have been used for thousands of years by many ancient civilizations to cleanse and exfoliate the skin. The Latin root *exfoliare* actually means to "strip off leaves." The Egyptians were considered the first to use the ritual practice of exfoliation for cleansing and purification, which was seen as a means to sustain life even into the afterworld.

The goal of many of the health and beauty treatments you'll learn about in this book has to do with some type of exfoliation practice. This can be achieved by physically scrubbing the skin with an abrasive type of exfoliant like a natural bristle brush, Celtic salt or sugar, or through using some chemical exfoliation process from ingredients such as essential oils, clay, sea salt and seaweed, which contain compounds known to actively loosen toxins.

Celtic Sea Salt

To ensure the essential oils are absorbed into the salts, it's now recommended that the oils are first added to 1 teaspoon unscented liquid soap, like Castile for example, or other unscented natural liquid soap, before adding to sea salts.

Celtic or grey salt, as it is sometimes referred to, is a "moist," unrefined sea salt found along the coastal regions of France. Its light grey to almost light purple color comes from the clay found in the salt flats.

Celtic salt is usually collected by hand using traditional Celtic methods. It has gained great popularity in recent years in the culinary world and is considered by many to be the best quality salt available in the world today.

You can purchase Celtic salt finely ground to use as table salt or for seasoning cuisine; however, for facial and body scrubs, get the plump, coarse-ground variety.

The moistness of the green clay found naturally in the Celtic sea salt allows for fast penetration of your pure essential oils, making it an excellent carrier for aromatic scents when using it in all your scented products.

Another remarkable feature of Celtic salt is how long the scent of your oils will last once absorbed and preserved by the salt, which acts as a carrier.

Though the Celtic salt has a slight, faint scent, it is worth considering for use as a carrier for your more expensive oils like rose and helichrysum. If you'd like to carry the pure scent of an oil or blend with you, as in the case of an appetite suppressant, you may want to keep the salt handy to use as needed. Clients tell me how much they love the steadfast company of their aromatherapy smelling salts.

Body Butters

Although skincare has been around since the dawn of mankind, body butters are a relatively recent addition to a healthy skincare regimen.

Body butter gives your skin a fresh and youthful appearance and has the ability to keep skin moisturized. Body butters also act as a protective barrier from a harsh or toxic environment.

You can choose different types of body butters to use in your recipes. The body butter carries the name of the nut or seed oil it is derived from. You can mix different body butters together as desired to get multiple benefits from one or more of the nuts or seeds.

Cocoa Butter: Made from the cocoa bean, cocoa butter smells like chocolate and is rich in antioxidants and nutrients. Cocoa butter is one of the most stable fats known and has a slow rancidity rate with a storage life of 2–5 years. Its smooth, velvety texture and pleasant aroma has made it a popular ingredient in many modern-day skincare products. Frequently recommended for prevention of stretch marks, cocoa butter is excellent for treating dry, chapped, cracked or burned skin and as a daily moisturizer to prevent dry, itchy skin and mouth sores.

Shea Butter: Widely used in the cosmetics industry, shea butter comes from the nut of the African shea tree, contains antioxidants as well as vitamins A and E and may have anti-inflammatory properties. Shea butter is used for its moisturizing properties to make skin and hair care products like lip gloss, skin moisturizer creams and hair conditioners.

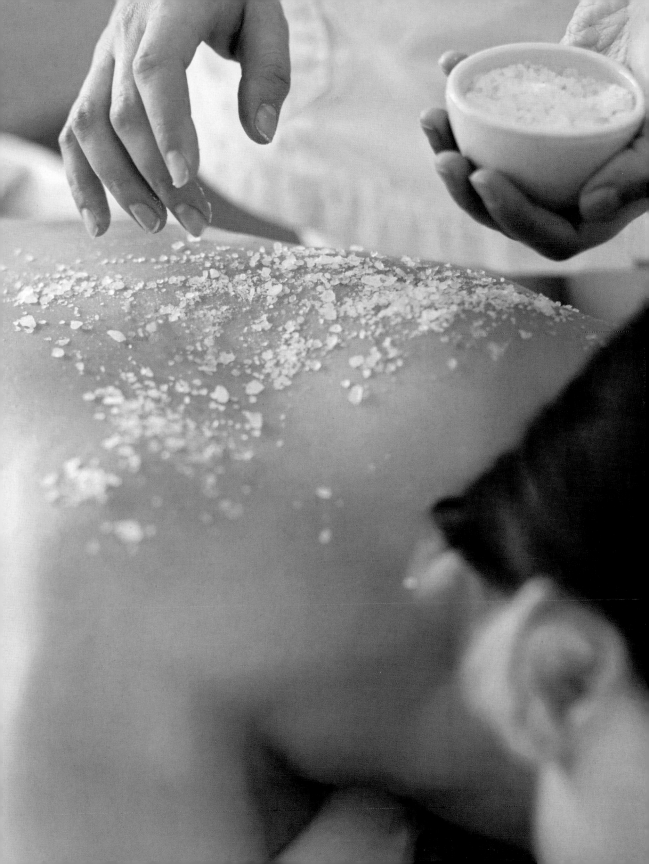

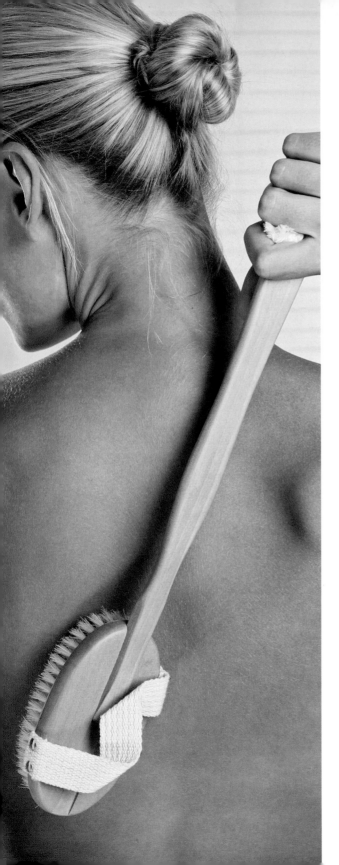

Beeswax: Although not a body butter, beeswax makes an excellent carrier for the soul-soothing scent of pure essential oil. I recommend using beeswax that is natural and unrefined as an ingredient in your body butter as needed. It will allow you to control the looseness or density of the body butter recipe you're creating. Beeswax can be used as a base for creams, balms, salves and lotions. The more beeswax you add to your recipe, the denser your product will be.

CAUTION: Many people have or can develop an allergy to nuts and seeds. It is a good idea to do a patch test with a new product before using it to make sure you do not have a reaction to it. If you have problems with excessively oily skin, the oils in body butters can aggravate the problem.

Skin Brushing

Skin brushing is one of the best ways to eliminate old, dead skin cell tissue and invigorate new skin growth. It keeps your skin healthy and glowing. As skin brushing stimulates your lymphatic system, it encourages detoxification. This cleansing and uplifting ritual of skin brushing is especially effective just before you shower.

You'll want to remember these key guidelines when skin brushing with a body brush for health:

- Always use a natural-bristle brush.
- Be gentle, yet brisk when brushing your skin, covering your entire body and omitting your face and neck in the process.
- Always be sure your brush strokes are from your extremities upward, toward your heart.
- Remember to breathe.
- Relax.

General Directions for Skin Body Brushing

1. Brush from your fingers up to your shoulders.

2. Brush from your toes up to your neck.

3. Include the front and back side of your body as you breathe deeply.

4. Enjoy the wonderful tingling sensations dancing across your skin.

Skin brushing the body with pure essential oil is known to have the following therapeutic effects:

- Invigorates skin.
- Detoxifies the body and mind.
- Stimulates the lymphatic system.
- Improves circulation.
- Exfoliates and regenerates skin tissue.
- Nourishes skin cell tissues.
- Imparts a radiant, healthy glow to your complexion.
- Smoothes and softens your skin.

Perfume Oil

Perfume oil is the number one way I use essential oil. I wear perfume oil continuously and frequently mix and match different ones to enjoy the bouquet of scent sensations I can create.

I prefer perfume oils that are made in a 10 percent to 50 percent dilution of pure essential oil to carrier oil. You can also make your perfume oils with alcohol spirits like vodka, though the scent of the essential oil is definitely altered when added to alcohol. Also, alcohol is itself very drying and can cause skin sensitivity for some.

My favorite perfume carrier oil is fractionated coconut oil. I love that it is non-greasy and absorbs quickly into my skin, carrying the therapeutic benefits of the oil directly into my blood stream. But mostly, I love the fact that light coconut oil has no scent of its own and will not interfere with the smell of the pure essential oil I am wearing. Check out the "Face Carrier Oils" section on page 25 to find out more about fractionated coconut oil.

Why Use Perfume Oil?

1. It is a completely natural product. With no additives or preservatives, you know the exact ingredients because you put them there.

2. There is seldom any concern with skin sensitivity or sensitization when using an essential oil diluted in carrier oil, except with "hot" oils. Check out the list of "hot" oils in the "Safe Use of Essential Oils" section on page 37.

3. It is an economical way to use essential oils, and perfume oil is an excellent way to extend your very expensive oils.

4. Perfume oil offers ease of use; carry it wherever you go.

5. You can add it to your sea salt for a luxurious and unforgettable bath experience.

6. It stabilizes the volatility of an essential oil, extending the life of an essential oil or blend.

7. You can enjoy experimenting and creating a variety of scent sensations.

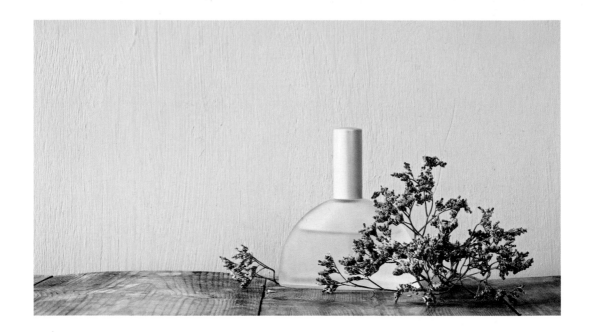

Aromatherapy Spray

An aromatherapy spray is another favorite way of mine to enjoy all the benefits of aromatic oils. Making your own personal aromatherapy spray is quick, simple and easy to do, as well as convenient to use.

You can make your own aromatherapy spray to use as a facial toner, an all-over body freshener or as a room spray and deodorizer. The amount of oil you use depends on the purpose of your aromatic mist.

Facial Toner: 6–10 drops. Shake well, mist onto a cotton facial pad and apply as facial toner.

Body Freshener: 6–10 drops. Shake well and lightly mist onto skin.

Air Freshener and Room Deodorizer: 120–180 drops. Shake well and mist into the air.

Start with a 2-ounce (60-ml) colored glass bottle with an atomizer (spray top). Fill halfway with approximately 600 drops of pure spring or purified water. Add your essential oil or blend. Fill the bottle with pure water, shake well and spray. The pure essential oils will float on top of the water, so you will need to shake your bottle to disperse the oils into the water each time before spraying. You may add an equal amount of alcohol or witch hazel (less drying than alcohol) to essential oils to act as a carrier for your oils to help keep them dispersed in the water. Remember, essential oils are very concentrated, and a little goes a long way.

PLEASE NOTE: Heavier oils can gum up the atomizer sprayer, especially the higher dilution amounts of oil. If this should happen, simply add more water to your atomizer bottle, shake well and spray.

CHAPTER 4

Safe Use
of Essential Oils

Never apply essential oils neat or undiluted on your skin. Always dilute your essential oils with a suitable vegetable carrier oil. I recommend cold processed, unfiltered or naturally filtered oils and preferably unscented, so you smell only your essential oil or blend of oils. Vegetable carrier oils like fractionated coconut oil or jojoba oil are both excellent choices. Stop using essential oils immediately if there is any skin irritation.

When using a pure, undiluted essential oil for inhalation, always keep a bottle of carrier oil, such as jojoba, handy. If pure essential oil comes in contact with your skin, dilute immediately with your carrier oil to avoid discomfort or possible skin irritation. Keep undiluted oils out of the reach of children.

Keep bottles of essential oils tightly closed and store them in a cool location away from light. If stored properly and unopened, most essential oils will maintain their potency for years; however, quicker evaporating citrus oils and conifers have a shorter shelf life because of oxidation, which causes them to lose therapeutic qualities. (See "Proper Storage of Essential Oils" [page 41] for more information.)

Essential oils should be used sparingly. Remember one drop of an essential oil equals about 1–4 cups (26–104 g) or more of dried plant matter.

Never smell essential oils straight out of the bottle. The reason for this is twofold. First, you don't want to overwhelm your olfactory senses with a large quantity of essential oil when smelling straight out of the bottle. The second reason, and most important, is that the orifice reducer may likely have old essential oil that has oxidized. You will not be smelling fresh oil, but rancid oil with no therapeutic benefit. It's always best to dispense a drop of oil on a smell strip and inhale to experience your oil.

Sensitization: Please use caution in applying essential oils to broken skin as this can cause severe irritation and may lead to an immune system reaction known as *sensitization*.

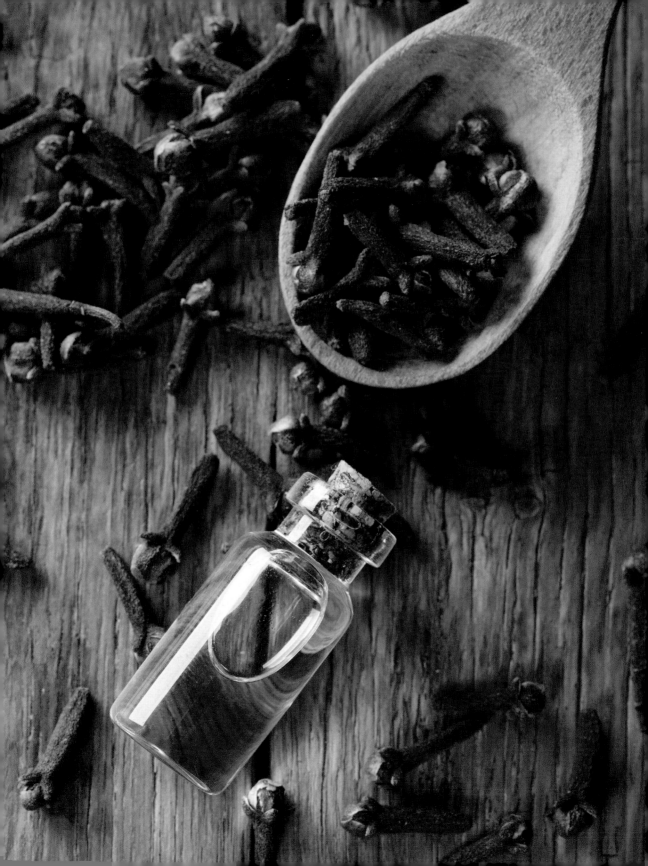

Skin sensitization is a type of allergic reaction that may occur when first exposed to an essential oil. However, in some instances, there may be little or no noticeable effect on the skin at the time of application, though exposure to the same or similar material in future applications may result in cross-sensitization and trigger a severe inflammatory reaction by the immune system. Skin reactions may appear as hot red welts, redness or rash, and can be quite painful to some individuals.

How to reduce the risk of sensitization

• Always properly dilute your essential oils within the recommended safety ranges (page 24). All essential oils have a maximum dilution rate set by the International Fragrance Association (www.ifraorg.org). These can also be found in Robert B. Tisserand's trusted reference book, *Essential Oil Safety.*
• Start with the lowest dilution percentage of essential oil to carrier and increase in small amounts.
• Avoid daily application of the same essential oil for prolonged periods of time.
• Avoid known sensitizers.
• Avoid using oxidized oils, especially from the Pinaceae family (such as pines and cypress species) and Rutaceae family (such as citrus oils).

Keep essential oils out of the reach of children. Handle and care for your essential oils as you would any product for therapeutic use.

Self-selection: When using essential oils in dilution with your child, I recommend you use self-selection. If your child gives any indication they dislike an aroma, the aroma is too strong. If there is any skin sensitivity, please discontinue use. You may dilute your essential oils further and try again at another time. Be respectful and allow your child to self-select.

Photosensitizing Oils: Avoid direct sunlight and essential oils. Some oils are known to be "photosensitizers." Most common are bergamot and other cold-pressed citrus oils. Photosensitizing oils should not be used on skin that will be exposed to sunlight or ultraviolet light for 4–6 hours or longer as this may increase your chance of sunburn and cause uneven skin pigmentation—also known as *berloque dermatitis.*

Essential oils rich in menthol (such as peppermint) should not be used on the throat or neck area of children under thirty months of age. Please note: Menthol is found in high concentrations of many over-the-counter pharmaceutical vapor rubs in common use for congestion.

Keep pure essential oils away from the eye area and do not put them into the ears.

Pregnant Women: Generally, I recommend exercising caution when using pure essential oils during the first trimester. Though if suffering from severe morning sickness early in pregnancy, the smell of peppermint or spearmint oil can be safe to use and may relieve the nausea. If the skin should become itchy or inflamed during pregnancy, please exercise caution as essential oils in massage or in the bath might make the condition worse.

Mothers of newborn babies should not use, or at least limit the use of, pure essential oils. One of the key reasons for this is because it can interfere with a mother's natural smell and thus interfere with the all-important bonding that occurs between a mother and her child.

Epileptics and people with high blood pressure should consult their health care professional before using essential oils. Avoid hyssop, fennel and wild tansy oils.

You may wish to skin test a small area first if you suffer from hay fever or allergies. Skin tests should always be done for very young children and the elderly.

Skin Test: Apply pure essential oil in a weak, 1 percent dilution of carrier oil on a cotton swab and lightly touch the skin in an area either under the arm, inside the elbow, behind the knee or on the wrist. Cover the area with a bandage and leave unwashed for 24 hours. If there is any reaction such as itching or redness, you may wish to discontinue using the oil. Sometimes a reaction to an essential oil can indicate a need for an internal cleansing program before using an essential oil. Essential oils can react with toxins built up in the body from chemicals in food, water and the environment. However, sensitivity can also simply be a sign that you are sensitive to one or more of the chemical properties in the essential oil, and you should not use that essential oil.

Hot Oils

Special care should be taken when using "hot" oils. Hot oils are those that have higher-than-usual potential for skin irritation and are often high in phenols, which contain carvacrol, eugenol and thymol compounds. Always use hot oils in extremely weak dilutions of less than 1 percent for skin application. Commonly used hot essential oils that may be potential skin irritants include:

- Basil (*Ocimum basilicum*)
- Black pepper (*Piper nigrum*)
- Cinnamon (*Cinnamomum zeylanicum*)
- Clove (*Eugenia caryophyllata*)
- Ginger (*Zingiber officinale*)
- Oregano (*Origanum vulgare*)
- Scotch pine (*Pinus sylvestris*)
- Siberian balsam (*Abies sibirica*)
- Silver fir (*Abies sibirica, alba, balsamea*)
- Thyme (*Thymus vulgaris*)
- Wintergreen (*Gaultheria procumbens*) *not recommended for use

In some cases:

- Tea tree (*Melaleuca alternifolia*)
- Ylang ylang (*Cananga odorata*)
- Peppermint (*Mentha x piperita*)

If any of these essential oils is applied in a weak dilution on the skin and a hot, red weal or skin reaction occurs, this is the result of skin irritation that requires immediate attention. Always have a vegetable carrier oil like pure fractionated coconut oil or jojoba available to apply onto the skin in such cases.

Applying carrier oil will have the immediate effect of calming the skin irritation. Do not wash or rinse the area with water as this will drive the essential oils further into the skin and increase, not diminish, the discomfort.

If you accidentally get essential oil in your eye, use a cotton tissue or swab at the corner of your eye to wick (absorb or draw out) the oil from the eye.

Essential oils are flammable. Please keep them out of the way of fire hazards.

Internal use: Essential oils should never be used internally for medicinal purposes without trained, professional medical guidance and direct supervision.

Essential oils are approved by the FDA and generally regarded as safe (GRAS) to use as food flavors. You can safely enjoy all the therapeutic effects of essential oils when using them as food flavors.

Proper Storage of Essential Oils

As essential oils are highly volatile and quickly evaporate when exposed to the air, care must be taken to store them properly. This means keeping your essential oils tightly sealed in dark-colored glass bottles. You want to store your oils in a cool, dark place, out of direct sunlight and out of the reach of children and animals. Artificial and fluorescent lighting can have a detrimental effect on essential oils and shorten their shelf life.

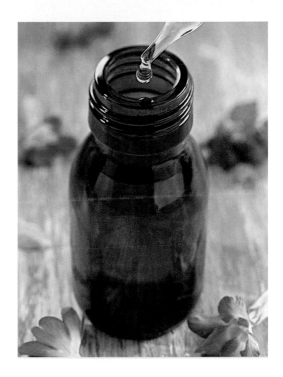

Pure essential oils will break down plastic and should never be stored undiluted in plastic bottles. Properly stored essential oils that have been sealed, unopened and kept in a cool, dark place will maintain their potency for many years.

The only exception to this may be the quicker evaporating citrus oils (such as grapefruit, orange, lime, mandarin and lemon) and conifers and firs (such as fir, pine and cypress). These oils have a shorter shelf life because high volatility leads to faster oxidation, causing them to lose any characteristic therapeutic properties, actions and effects.

Citrus oils are by far the most volatile of all the essential oils. Special care needs to be taken to keep them tightly sealed and stored in a darkened area that is both dry and cool. You can limit the amount of oxidation of your essential oils by keeping them in bottles that are filled to capacity in which there is no room inside the bottle for oxidation to occur.

You can consider refrigerating your citrus oils, blue oils, conifers and others to increase shelf life as long as the oils are kept in a dry condition and are stored for long-term use rather than being dispensed daily. Refrigerating your blue oils will help them retain their vibrant blue color. Never refrigerate rose oil, as it will thicken and congeal. Thicker, viscous oils have a low volatility rate and, as long as the bottle is filled to capacity, will have a very slow oxidation rate.

Shelf Life for Essential Oils

Many things can affect the shelf life of an essential oil. This is a general guide for a short list of essential oils. Proper storage can significantly increase the longevity of an oil's shelf life and its therapeutic quality. If an oil is stored in a dark, glass bottle that is filled to capacity and kept sealed, this guide will give you a general idea about shelf life.

Note: If an essential oil begins to appear cloudy, thicken or smell more acidic, it has likely begun to oxidize.

Approximately 6 months–2 or 3 years from date of distillation:

- Bay Laurel (*Laurus nobilis*)
- Cypress (*Cupressus sempervirens*)
- Eucalyptus* (*Eucalyptus globulus* and *radiata*)
- Fir Needle (*Abies concolor*)
- Frankincense (*Boswellia frereana*)
- Grapefruit (*Citrus paradisi*)
- Juniper Berry (*Juniperus communis*)
- Lemon (*Citrus limonum*)
- Lemongrass (West Indian) (*Cymbopogon citratus*)
- Lime (*Citrus aurantifolia*)
- Mandarin (*Citrus deliciosa*)
- Nutmeg (*Myristica fragrans*)
- Sweet Orange (*Citrus sinensis*)
- Petitgrain (*Citrus aurantium*)
- Pine (*Abies sibirica*)
- Black Spruce (*Picea mariana*)
- Tangerine (*Citrus reticulata*)

*If stored properly and/or refrigerated, eucalyptus can last up to 5 years.

Approximately 3–4 years from date of distillation:

- Ammi Visnaga (Khella Plant Seeds) (*Ammi Visnaga*)
- Black Pepper (*Piper nigrum*)
- Bergamot (*Citrus bergamia*)
- Carrot Seed (*Daucus carota*)
- Cinnamon Leaf (*Cinnamomum zeylanicum*)
- Clove Bud (*Eugenia caryophyllata*)
- Eucalyptus (*Eucalyptus globulus* and *radiata*)
- Fennel, Bitter (*Foeniculum vulgare*)
- Helichrysum (*Helichrysum italicum*)
- Ledum (*Ledum groenlandicum*)
- Myrtle (*Myrtus communis*)
- Naiouli (*Melaleuca quinquenervia*)
- Neroli (*Citrus aurantium var amara*)

Approximately 4–5 years from date of distillation:

- Basil (*Ocimum basilicum*, ct linalool)
- Clary Sage (*Salvia sclarea*)
- Eucalyptus (*Eucalyptus globulus* and *radiata*)
- Geranium (*Pelargonium graveolens* and *roseum*)
- German Chamomile (*Matricaria recutita*)
- Ginger (*Zingiber officinale*)
- Lavender (*Lavandula angustifolia*)
- Palmarosa (*Cymbopogon martinii*)
- Peppermint (*Mentha x piperita*)
- Roman Chamomile (*Anthemis nobilis*)
- Ylang Ylang (*Cananga odorata*)

Approximately 6–8 years from date of distillation:

- Cedarwood (*Cedrus atlantica* or *deodora*)
- Myrrh (*Commiphora myrrha*)
- Patchouli (*Pogostemon cablin*)
- Sandalwood (*Santalum album*)
- Vetiver (*Vetiveria zizanioides*)

CHAPTER 5

Aromatherapy Supplies

What You Need to Have on Hand for Making Your Products

This is the shopping list of aromatherapy supplies I suggest you have on hand. You will learn about the therapeutic use of each of the oils, as well as how to use them in formulating your own therapeutic blends and aromatherapy treatments.

When selecting pure essential oils, the minimal requirements for choosing your oils should include:

1. Generic name of the essential oil.

2. Botanical species of the plant.

3. Part of the plant that produced the oil.

4. Method of extraction used.

5. Location where the oil was produced.

Bergamot (*Citrus bergamia*): cold-pressed peel, Italy

Eucalyptus (*globulus* and *radiata*): steam-distilled leaf, Australia

Frankincense (*Boswellia frereana*): steam-distilled resin tears, Somalia

Geranium Roseum and Graveolens (*Pelargonium roseum* and *graveolens*): steam-distilled leaves, Madagascar and Albania

Helichrysum (*Helichrysum italicum, Immortelle*): steam-distilled flowers, Italy

Lavender (*Lavandula angustifolia*): steam-distilled flowers, High Altitude France, Bulgaria or Italy

Lemon (*Citrus limonum*): cold-pressed peel, Italy

Peppermint (*Mentha x piperita*): steam-distilled flowering tops, USA

Roman Chamomile (*Chamaemelum nobile*): steam-distilled flower, USA and France

Sweet Marjoram (*Origanum marjorana*): steam-distilled flowers and leaf, Egypt (page 45)

Tea Tree (*Melaleuca alternifolia*): steam-distilled leaf, Australia (page 45)

Vetiver (*Vetiveria zizanioides*): hydrodiffused root, Haiti

Ylang Ylang (*Cananga odorata*): steam-distilled flowers, Madagascar (page 45)

Supplemental Oils to Have on Hand for Concocting Aromatherapy Formulations

Very expensive oils like rose can be purchased in a 10 percent dilution of carrier oil. The intensity of these pure oils makes them useful in dilution with great effect.

Ammi Visnaga (*Ammi visnaga*): steam-distilled herb, Morocco

Atlas Cedarwood (*Cedrus atlantica*): steam-distilled wood, Morocco (endangered)

Black Pepper (*Piper nigrum*): steam-distilled fruit, Madagascar

Black Spruce (*Picea mariana*): steam-distilled needle, Canada (page 45)

Carrot Seed (*Daucus carota*): steam-distilled seed, France (page 45)

Cinnamon (*Cinnamomum zeylanicum*): steam-distilled leaf, Madagascar (page 45)

Clove (*Eugenia caryophyllata*): steam-distilled bud, Madagascar

Cypress (*Cupressus sempervirens*): steam-distilled leaf, Crete

German Chamomile (*Matricaria chamomilla*): steam-distilled flower, Bulgaria (page 45)

Ginger (*Zingiber officinale*): hydrodiffused fresh root, Sri Lanka and Madagascar

Hyssop (*Hyssopus officinalis*): steam-distilled whole plant, Bulgaria

Ledum (*Ledum groenlandicum*): steam-distilled herb, Canada (page 45)

Melissa (*Melissa officinalis*): steam-distilled flowers and leaves, England and France (page 45)

Myrrh (*Commiphora myrrha*): steam-distilled gum resin, Ethiopia (the BEST) and Somalia

Neroli (*Citrus aurantium*): steam-distilled flower, Tunisia

Oregano (*Origanum vulgare*): steam-distilled herb, Turkey

Palmarosa (*Cymbopogon martinii*): steam-distilled herb, Nepal

Patchouli (*Pogostemon cablin*): steam-distilled leaf, Indonesia (page 45)

Red Mandarin (*Citrus deliciosa*): cold-pressed peel, Italy

Rosemary (*Rosmarinus officinalis ct. verbenone* and *cineole*): steam-distilled flowering herb and leaf, Italy

Rose Otto (*Rosa damascena*): steam-distilled flowers, Turkey and Bulgaria

Sandalwood (*Santalum album*): steam-distilled heartwood, Mysore, India (endangered) (page 45)

Sweet Orange (*Citrus sinensis*): cold-pressed fresh peel, Italy

Thyme (*Thymus vulgaris*): steam-distilled herb, Germany and France

Yarrow (*Achillea millefolium*): steam-distilled flower, Bulgaria (page 45)

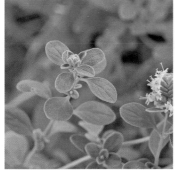

Sweet Marjoram (*Origanum marjorana*)

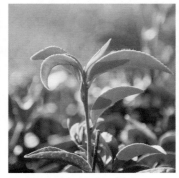

Tea Tree (*Melaleuca alternifolia*)

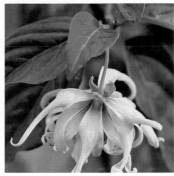

Ylang Ylang (*Cananga odorata*)

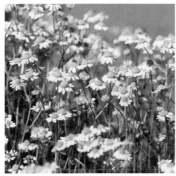

Black Spruce (*Picea mariana*)

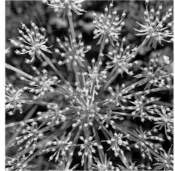

Carrot Seed (*Daucus carota*)

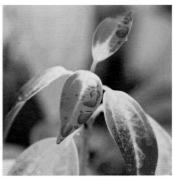

Cinnamon (*Cinnamomum zeylanicum*)

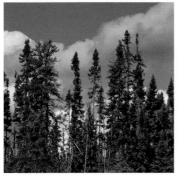

German Chamomile (*Matricaria chamomilla*)

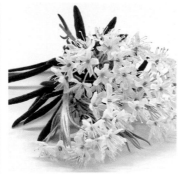

Ledum (*Ledum groenlandicum*)

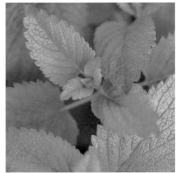

Melissa (*Melissa officinalis*)

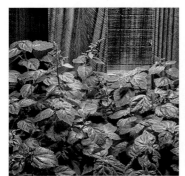

Patchouli (*Pogostemon cablin*)

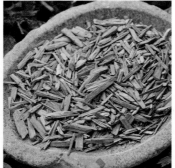

Sandalwood (*Santalum album*)

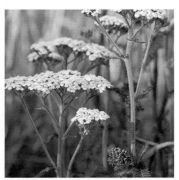

Yarrow (*Achillea millefolium*)

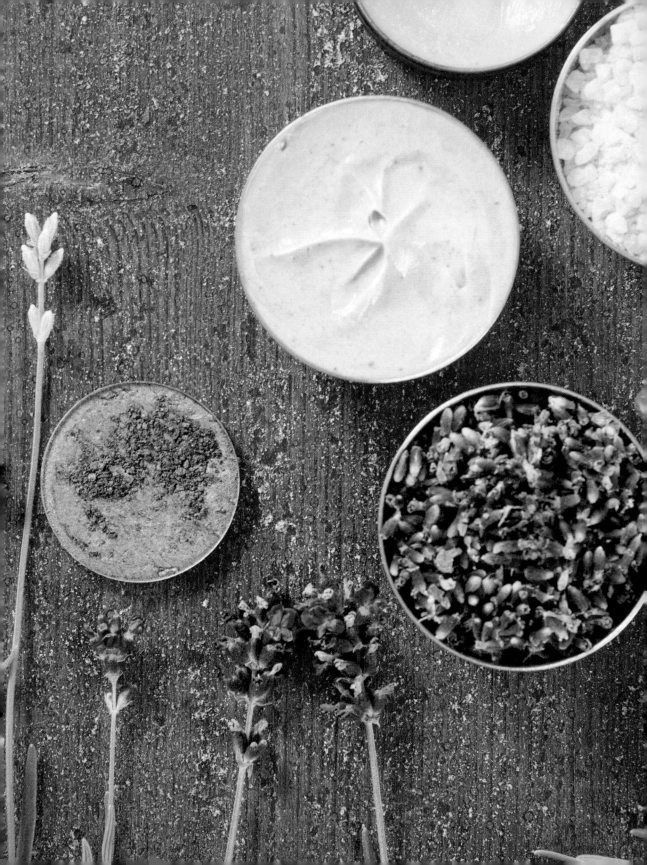

Additional Supplies to Consider Having On Hand

- Seven 1-ounce (30-ml) bottles of vegetable carrier oil (for making aromatic medicine and blends)
- Ten 5-milliliter, colored-glass, euro-dropper bottles (for making aromatic medicine and blends)
- 1 bag cotton balls
- 1 packet smell strips
- Natural bristle skin brush
- Cotton washcloth
- Cotton hand towel
- Cotton bath towel
- Robe

Aromatherapy Journal: Highly recommended for recording personal notes about your experiences with essential oils, as well as the various recipes and blends you formulate.

As some of the pure essential oils are very expensive, you may wish to buy them in a 10 percent dilution to use in your aromatherapy products. Please be sure to add a 10 percent dilution of an oil directly to your carrier before application, not to a synergy blend as they will not synergize with the other essential oils.

For Making Aromatherapy Sprays

- 2 or more 2-ounce (60-ml) colored-glass atomizer misting bottles
- 1 quart (945 ml), or more, purified water
- Optional: Witch hazel or alcohol

For Making Smelling Salts

- ¼ cup (130 g) Celtic (grey) salt
- ⅛-ounce (4-ml) vial(s) with cap for smelling salts

For Making Aromatic Bath Salts

- Sea salt
- Epsom salts
- Celtic (grey) salts
- Baking soda

For Making Facial and Body Masks and Scrubs

- 1 cup (200 g) sugar
- 1 cup (236 ml) honey
- 1 cup (236 ml) cream
- 1 cup (230 g) French green or pink clay
- 1 avocado
- 1 egg

For Making Lip Balms, Butters, Creams, Healing Salves and Ointments

- 1 or more ¼- or ½-ounce (7- or 15-ml) colored-glass jars with lid
- One 4-ounce (118-ml) colored-glass jar with lid
- One 2-ounce (60-ml) colored-glass jar with lid
- ¼ cup (57 g), or more, beeswax
- Light coconut oil
- ¼ cup (55 g) shea butter
- Aloe vera gel
- Vegetable glycerin

For Facial and Respiratory Steams

- Stainless steel or ceramic bowl

For Aromatherapy Blends

- 1 dozen or more 5-milliliter, colored-glass, euro-dropper bottles

Optional Supplies

- Footbath or basin for foot soak
- Diffuser
- Humidifier

CHAPTER 6

Aromatherapy Blending Guide
(and Secrets)

I've always had a passion for music. There are a lot of analogies between aromatherapy blending and music. Formulating an essential oil blend is very much like making music. Like music, you can create essential oil blends that are very inspiring and uplifting to your senses that help you to relax and unwind, relieve cold and flu symptoms and more.

Your taste in music is often reflected in the aromas you love most and the blends you feel inspired to create. If you like hot, spicy salsa music, you are probably attracted to hot and spicy oils. If you like music that's relaxing, you're probably drawn to calming oils. Maybe you like a combination of both relaxing and stimulating oils depending upon the circumstances and your desired results.

I love music everywhere except in my blending room. For me, blending is very much a meditative experience. I usually like to blend in silence with no distractions, so that I can completely focus on creating my blend.

I also use biodynamic blending methods that take into consideration phases of the moon, among other things. Just like how the best days for planting are noted in the farmer's almanac, there are best times to create your blends.

Music and blending have in common both craftsmanship and artistry. You have to learn how to touch and be touched by the oils. It's very much an intimate relationship that you develop with the oils. I've always had this intuitive sense with essential oils. Some oils speak to me more loudly than others, but there is always a communion and partnership at the heart of my experience when blending oils.

Just like the finest culinary chefs with food ingredients or the most gifted musicians with their instruments, it's through developing an intimate relationship with the oils that you will learn how to create the greatest beauty and harmony when blending aromatic formulas. When you commune with your essential oils, you can produce incredible healing results in practice.

In aromatherapy, blending becomes craftsmanship when you learn how to use the tools of essential oils for healing. Craftsmanship is learning which essential oils to use for producing certain therapeutic results and discovering the method of application to use for the best outcomes and desired effects. When you learn the different techniques to use in practice, this is craftsmanship. Your craftsmanship allows the oils to achieve their greatest potential for promoting balance and healing.

Whereas artistry is when you're capturing the aromatic scents, creating harmony between ingredients and having those aromas enhance one another in a synergetic dance that is captivating to the senses.

Essential oils are not really tangible. They are aromatic vapors that quickly evaporate when they meet the elements of light, heat and air. Interestingly, it is the contact with the elements that releases the scent of essential oils. You actually feel aromatic scents. Your rational brain is not at all involved in your process of smell. Scent reaches the deepest part of you!

Just as with music, there are top or high notes, middle notes and bottom or base notes. You want to create a blend of oils that can become like music, harmonious and pleasing to your senses, all while having the qualities needed to produce the desired therapeutic effects. When you make music with essential oils it moves beyond craftsmanship to artistry and becomes a visceral experience.

To keep your blends vibrant and consistent you have to use all your knowledge and the blending techniques you will learn. You will also need to connect with your blend exactly like a musician does to make music so that you and others can appreciate and benefit from using your essential oil blend.

My blending secrets will guide you step-by-step in exactly how to create the perfect blend. You will learn how to wed the artistry of blending with the craftsmanship needed to make each of your blends sing and achieve remarkable results.

After a little practice, you will know the aroma qualities and effects of many different essential oils and enjoy creating your very own aromatherapy blends to satisfy your personal needs!

To make a blend of essential oils for the first time, I recommend you start with a bottle that is larger than necessary so you have room to experiment and allow your blend to evolve. When I create a new blend, I usually start with a 1-ounce (30-ml) colored-glass bottle that can be tightly sealed with a screw cap.

You're experimenting with the oils to create your perfect blend, and it's best to have plenty of room to formulate your blend. Later you can transfer your blend to a smaller colored-glass, euro-dropper bottle for dispensing your oils. Right now you're in the blending creation mode.

Next you must decide for what purpose you want to use your essential oil blend. Is it a perfume or pain-relief oil, or is it for relaxation, beauty or skincare?

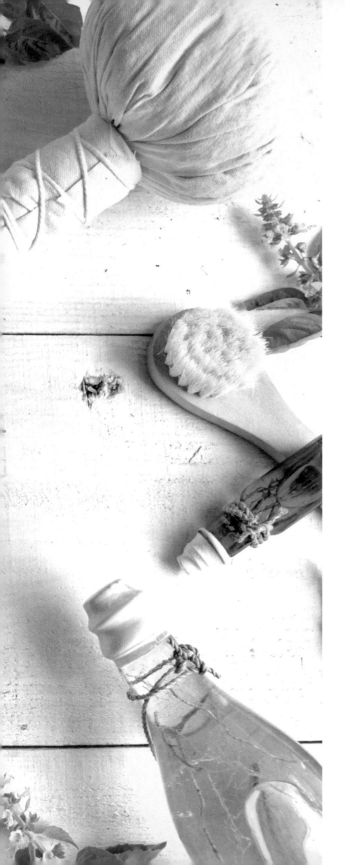

Essential Oil Blending Directions

1. Choose three essential oils (top, middle and base notes) you want to use in your blend.

2. Use an aromatherapy journal or a clean sheet of paper to write down the names of each essential oil you will be using to formulate your blend. You will record the number of drops of each oil you add to your blend. You will be writing down the recipe that you're creating.

3. Add 1–3 drops of your selected essential oil. Write down its aroma quality and characteristic effects and whether it is a top, middle or base note.

   I like to start with base notes as they are less volatile and will not have an immediate tendency to evaporate. The base note will also anchor the middle and high notes, so they're less susceptible to rapid evaporation. If you're going to walk away from your blend for any length of time, I recommend you cap the bottle tightly as a precaution to prevent evaporation. This also helps you develop your relationship with the oils. For me, aromatic blending is a sacred act of communion with the oils, and I'm always sending them my love and appreciation.

4. Add 1–3 drops of another of your selected essential oils. Write down its aroma quality and characteristic effects and whether it's a top, middle or base note.

5. Add 1–3 drops of your third essential oil, noting its aroma quality and characteristic effects, as well as if it is a top, middle or base note.

6. Cap the top of the bottle and shake vigorously, blending the oils.

Now it's time to sample your blend's aroma.

Dispense one drop onto a smell strip, tissue or cotton ball and inhale the aroma of your blend. When sampling the aroma, you will probably notice the scent of one of the essential oils more than the rest. This is usually the case. The lighter, higher top notes are usually most discernible.

As your blend begins to synergize, the aroma qualities will change and take on a unique character. Allow space for this synergistic action to happen. You'll be glad you did. How you begin sets a firm foundation for your blend. You're gathering the information you need to create a truly mesmerizing blend. So take time for your blend to synergize.

Writing down your aroma experiences deepens your awareness of each essential oil and how it blends with other oils.

At a certain point, usually within 30 minutes, but sometimes longer, you'll notice the blend's aroma begins to stabilize. One of the reasons I use only 3–9 drops when first making a blend is that less time for synergy is required.

You will notice that the aroma of certain essential oils lingers longer in your memory.

Are you able to discern the individual oils? How have the oils changed or been enhanced by the other oils in the blend? Write down everything you notice about your experience of the three blended oils.

Now the next important question to answer is are you happy with the ratio of the oils? Does 1–3 drops of each oil in the blend seem the right ratio? Or, does your blend lack harmony?

The aromatic qualities and the language of aromas sing to your senses like muses inspiring you to formulate a balanced blend for harmonizing body, mind, spirit and emotions. Listen deeply as you experiment with your aromatic formulation. As you do this you will naturally get a feel for when to emphasize a particular aromatic note. You will begin to understand the language of aroma to achieve your desired results.

Then add one additional drop of any one of the oils that especially called to you. You may feel that you want to experience more of that particular note in your blend. Be sure to record each drop you add to your blend in your journal or on your recipe sheet.

Mix the blend again and inhale. Follow the above guidelines for allowing your blend to synergize, and take time to fully experience it before moving forward. Take time to formulate your recipe slowly in gradual steps. Focus and pay close attention. Continue to notice and note your experience of the oils as you create your blend.

Continue to add one drop at a time of any of the oils that calls to you until you feel the blend is complete and pleases your senses.

Keeping track of the number of drops of each essential oil while blending ensures you won't forget the exact recipe of a blend should it be a memorable one for you.

CHAPTER 7

Aromatherapy
Formulas

After experimenting with creating your own essential oil blend, try these three types of starter aromatherapy blends. Allow your blend to synergize for at least 30 minutes, then pour your blend into a 1-ounce (30-ml) bottle of your favorite carrier oil in the recommended dilution amounts given for each blend.

1% Dilution — Headache Relief Blend (9–15 drops total)

- Eucalyptus, *Eucalyptus globulus*: 2 drops
- Peppermint, *Mentha x piperita*: 3 drops
- Lavender, *Lavandula angustifolia*: 4 drops

2% Dilution — Immune Stimulant Blend (15–18 drops total)

- Lavender, *Lavandula angustifolia*: 5 drops
- Manuka, *Leptospermum scoparium*: 5 drops
- Eucalyptus, *Eucalyptus radiata*: 5 drops

5% Dilution — Sore Muscle Blend (30–45 drops total)

- Marjoram, *Origanum majorana*: 10 drops
- Peppermint, *Mentha x piperita*: 10 drops
- Lavender, *Lavandula angustifolia*: 10 drops

Rub a little of your Headache Relief or Immune Stimulant essential oil blend diluted in carrier oil on your wrists, your temples or the sides of your neck or chest. Try the Sore Muscle Blend on a tense muscle or painful joint.

Use your blend several times at intervals over the next several days and notice what effect it has on you. Share your blend with family and friends, and ask them to report any effects they notice and how they enjoyed the oil. Make notes about all of your observations and how others who use the blend respond.

Also, notice if your essential oil blend changes over time. Does the scent of your blend smell the same on a smell strip as when applied to your skin? Or is it somehow different?

By trying out your essential blends with others and using different methods of application you are learning valuable information for creating essential oil blends that heal. Through exploring the uses and benefits of essential oils you will become confident about using them in your everyday life.

Next, try the following essential oil blends to test out your skills.

Massage Oil Blends

An aromatherapy massage has been shown to have therapeutic effects to calm your mind and emotions. It can also be used to promote muscle pain relief, speed healing of injuries and aid recovery from illness, physically demanding work and rigorous exercise.

An 8-month study was conducted on eight subjects who were given a weekly aromatherapy massage for 6 weeks. Each subject's level of anxiety and depression was measured using the Hospital Anxiety and Depression Scale (HADS) prior to their first massage and again after their final massage. Improvements were reported in six out of the eight test subjects.

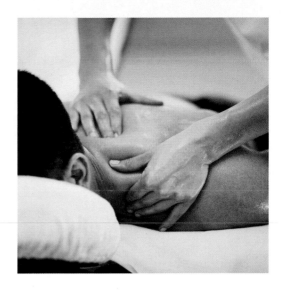

Relaxation Formula

This formula is perfect as your go-to blend or for the beginner who is new to the world of aromatherapy massage. Always pleasing!

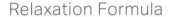

To a 5-ml euro-dropper bottle add:

Vetiver: 20 drops

Cypress: 20 drops

Lavender: 20 drops

Clary Sage: 10 drops

Bergamot: 30 drops

Close the cap tightly and shake the bottle vigorously to thoroughly blend the essential oils. Allow to synergize for 8 or more hours before using.

To make a ready-to-use relaxation blend, simply add 15–30 drops of your synergy blend to a 1-ounce (30-ml) bottle of your favorite carrier oil. Shake the bottle well to disperse the oils thoroughly. Use as a massage oil lubricant.

Sports Injury Formula

If you, a friend, a loved one or a client has an injury, especially one involving soft tissue, muscles, ligaments or tendons, this is a great blend you can rely on to speed healing and recovery.

To a 5-ml euro-dropper bottle add:

Sweet Marjoram: 40 drops

Helichrysum: 10 drops

Cypress: 40 drops

Peppermint: 10 drops

Close the cap tightly and shake the bottle vigorously to thoroughly blend the essential oils. Allow to synergize for 8 or more hours before using.

To make a ready-to-use sports injury blend, simply add 15–30 drops of your synergy blend to a 1-ounce (30-ml) bottle of your favorite carrier oil. Shake the bottle well to disperse the oils thoroughly. Use as a massage oil lubricant.

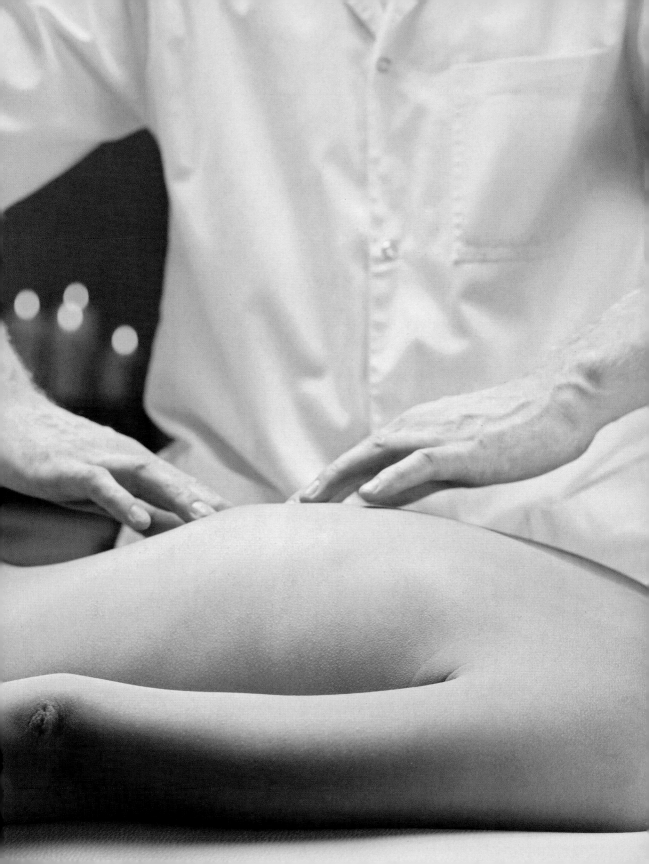

Calming Formula

When you need a blend that will help to ease and soothe an overly active or agitated mind and emotions, this is the blend to use.

To a 5-ml euro-dropper bottle add:

Lavender: 20 drops

Sweet Marjoram: 20 drops

Ylang Ylang III: 20 drops

Roman Chamomile: 20 drops

Red Mandarin: 20 drops

Close the cap tightly and shake the bottle vigorously to thoroughly blend the essential oils. Allow to synergize for 8 or more hours before using.

To make a ready-to-use calming blend, simply add 15–30 drops of your synergy blend to a 1-ounce (30-ml) bottle of your favorite carrier oil. Shake the bottle well to disperse the oils thoroughly. Use as a massage oil lubricant.

Restorative Formula

When your energy feels low, or you feel run-down or overly tired from not enough rest or sleep, or because you've been burning the candle at both ends, use this restorative formula. It will give your energy a boost, as well as freshen your thoughts and emotions and get you going in the right direction.

To a 5-ml euro-dropper bottle add:

Myrrh: 40 drops

Frankincense: 40 drops

Lemongrass: 10 drops

Galbanum: 1–2 drops

Black Spruce: 10 drops

Close the cap tightly and shake the bottle vigorously to thoroughly blend the essential oils. Allow to synergize for 8 or more hours before using.

To make a ready-to-use restorative blend, simply add 15–30 drops of your synergy blend to a 1-ounce (30-ml) bottle of your favorite carrier oil. Shake the bottle well to disperse the oils thoroughly. Use as a massage oil lubricant.

Muscle Pain Relief Formula

When your body feels sore and aches, this is a great oil you can rely on to ease your pain and give you the desired relief. It's also refreshing and restorative to your mind and emotions.

To a 5-ml euro-dropper bottle add:

Sweet Marjoram: 80 drops

Ginger: 10 drops

Peppermint: 10 drops

Close the cap tightly and shake the bottle vigorously to thoroughly blend the essential oils. Allow to synergize for 8 or more hours before using.

To make a ready-to-use muscle pain relief blend, simply add 15–30 drops of your synergy blend to a 1-ounce (30-ml) bottle of your favorite carrier oil. Shake the bottle well to disperse the oils thoroughly. Use as a massage oil lubricant.

CHAPTER 8

Healing *Blends*

These blends will help you become more aware of how aromatherapy works as you continue to practice the art. Feel your confidence grow and bring relief to yourself and others with these Healing Blends.

Headache Relief Formula 1

Headache is the most common form of physical pain. More than 50 percent of adults in the U.S. will experience some kind of headache this year. Symptoms of a headache may include pain in the head and neck regions, loss of appetite, poor sleep, light headedness and dizziness. Headaches may be caused by many different conditions such as dehydration, toxicity in the body, cold and flu, head injury, structural deviations of the neck, dental and sinus issues, sleep deprivation, food allergies and intolerances, and medications, among others. There are three main types of headaches experienced: migraines, tension headaches and cluster headaches. Commonly, the method of treatment used most often for headache is pain medication that can have unwanted side effects.

The essential oils in this Headache Relief Formula have been shown to be effective for relieving symptoms of tension and migraine headaches. The blend contains powerful analgesic pain relievers, vasoconstrictors and decongestants that promote circulation and shrink swollen membranes. The formula works best if used immediately at the first sign of a headache.

Tension and migraine headaches may be a sign of dehydration. Be sure to drink plenty of pure, fresh water daily. The guideline for sufficient water intake is generally half your body weight in ounces daily.

To a 5-ml, colored-glass, euro-dropper bottle add:

Peppermint: 20 drops

Marjoram: 20 drops

Eucalyptus: 20 drops

Lavender: 20 drops

Lemon: 10 drops

Juniper Berry: 5 drops

Basil: 5 drops

Cap the bottle tightly and shake vigorously to blend the essential oils. Allow to synergize for 8 hours or longer before using.

Dispense 1–3 drops on a cotton ball or smell strip and inhale the aromatic vapors of your headache relief blend for 10–15 seconds. You may repeat as needed. The formula is also effective when diffused into the air or used as a cool compress applied to the back of your neck.

To make a ready-to-use headache relief blend simply add 15–30 drops of your synergy blend to a 1-ounce (30-ml) bottle of your favorite carrier oil. Shake the bottle well to disperse the oils thoroughly. Apply a few drops of your ready-to-use headache relief blend to sinus points around your nose and forehead, as well as on the back of your neck.

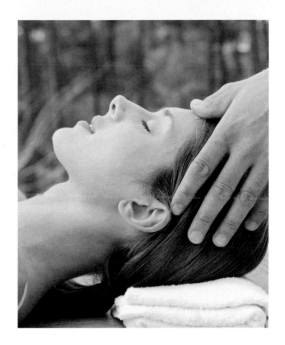

Headache Relief Formula 2

A second headache relief formula to try. It contains the same analgesics and vasoconstrictors with a more gentle feel when using. It promotes circulation and shrinking of swollen membranes. It's best if used at the first signs of headache.

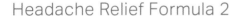

To a 5-ml, colored-glass, euro-dropper bottle add:
Peppermint: 30 drops
Sweet Marjoram: 30 drops
Lavender: 10 drops
Eucalyptus: 30 drops

Close the cap tightly and shake the bottle vigorously to thoroughly blend the essential oils. Allow to synergize for 8 or more hours before using.

Dispense 1–3 drops on a cotton ball or smell strip and inhale the aromatic vapors of your headache relief blend for 10–15 seconds. You may repeat as needed. This formula may also be effective as a cool compress.

To make a ready-to-use headache relief blend, simply add 15–30 drops of your synergy blend to a 1-ounce (30-ml) bottle of your favorite carrier oil. Shake the bottle well to disperse the oils thoroughly. Apply a few drops of your ready-to-use headache relief blend to sinus points around your nose and forehead, as well as on the back of your neck. Best results are obtained when you use your headache relief blend at the first signs of a headache. Clients report that with regular use their headaches diminish in severity, are less frequent or seemed to stop altogether.

Migraine Relief Formula

About 15 percent of the world's population experiences migraines. A migraine is a recurring type of primary headache that affects half of the head with throbbing pain that lasts for up to 72 hours. Associated symptoms, which may be mild to intense, include nausea, vomiting and sensitivity to movement, light, heat, sound and smell. Most people report having an aura before a migraine episode, which is a visual cue that signals a migraine is about to occur.

Thought to be caused by a combination of both genetic and environmental influences, migraines may be inherited through one's family of origin. Changing hormone levels may also play a role as the fluctuation increases pressure on the blood vessels and nerves of the brain, resulting in a migraine.

The essential oils in this formula have been shown to be effective as a comfort care measure for relieving the painful symptoms associated with a migraine headache.

To a 5-ml, colored-glass, euro-dropper bottle add:
Peppermint: 40 drops
Lavender: 20 drops
Cypress: 20 drops
Frankincense: 20 drops

Close the cap tightly and shake the bottle vigorously to thoroughly blend the essential oils. Allow to synergize for 8 or more hours before using.

Dispense 1–3 drops on a cotton ball or smell strip and inhale the aromatic vapors of your migraine relief blend for 10–15 seconds. You may repeat as needed. This formula may also be effective as a cool compress.

To make a ready-to-use headache relief blend, simply add 15–30 drops of your synergy blend to a 1-ounce (30-ml) bottle of your favorite carrier oil. Shake the bottle well to disperse the oils thoroughly. Apply a few drops of your ready-to-use migraine relief blend to sinus points around your nose and forehead, as well as on the back of your neck. Best results are obtained when you use your migraine relief blend at the first signs of a migraine. Clients report that with regular use their migraines diminish in severity, are less frequent or seemed to stop altogether.

Pain Relief Formula

Research shows that pain, and the suffering it brings, is the number one driving force behind the alternative and complementary health care movement. As humans, we all seek to move toward pleasure and away from pain. These are the two forces that drive all human behavior.

Physical pain is an unpleasant sensation that may involve damage to tissues, or can also be experienced emotionally. No one likes to experience pain and will do whatever necessary to move away from it. Whether your pain is acute (short-term) or chronic (long-term), essential oils can help to provide symptomatic relief, as well as promote natural healing.

The essential oils in this comfort care formula may be effective for relieving symptoms of physical pain and the accompanying emotional discomfort.

To a 5-ml, colored-glass, euro-dropper bottle add:

Peppermint: 20 drops

Helichrysum: 20 drops

Sweet Marjoram: 20 drops

Ylang Ylang III: 10 drops

German Chamomile: 30 drops

Cap the bottle tightly and shake vigorously to blend the essential oils. Allow to synergize for 8 hours or longer before using.

Dispense 1–3 drops on a cotton ball or smell strip and inhale the aromatic vapors of your blend for 10–15 seconds. You may repeat as needed. This formula is also effective when diffused into the air.

To make a ready-to-use massage blend, simply add 15–30 drops of your synergy blend to a 1-ounce (30-ml) bottle of your favorite carrier oil. Shake the bottle well to disperse the oils thoroughly. Dispense 1–3 drops. Inhale the scent first and then gently apply a few drops of your ready-to-use blend to the area of pain and massage in thoroughly.

Muscle Pain Relief Formula

The medical term for muscle pain is *myalgia*. It is a common symptom in many disease processes, though commonly it's most often associated with chronic tension, overuse, over-stretching, injury, strain to a muscle or group of muscles and trauma. Muscle pain is also common to those who suffer with chronic fatigue syndrome.

To a 5-ml, colored-glass, euro-dropper bottle add:

Cypress: 30 drops

Sweet Marjoram: 35 drops

Ylang Ylang III: 10 drops

Lavender: 10 drops

Lemongrass: 5 drops

Peppermint: 5 drops

Helichrysum: 5 drops

Close the cap tightly and shake the bottle vigorously to thoroughly blend the essential oils. Allow to synergize for 8 or more hours before using.

Add 15–18 drops of your synergy blend to a 1-ounce (30-ml) bottle of your favorite carrier oil. Shake the bottle well to disperse the oils thoroughly. Apply a few drops and massage in to relieve strained or sore muscles, ligaments and tendons. Taking a hot shower or bath before applying will increase blood flow to enhance your results. Applying just before bed can be helpful for promoting deep and restful sleep, as well as supporting deep healing and recovery. It may also be effective as a hot compress.

Nerve Pain Relief Formula

The medical term for nerve pain is *neuralgia*. Neuralgia is a form of chronic pain that occurs when there is damage to a nerve. It is characterized by sharp, shooting pain that can be intermittent or ongoing. Nerve pain is often associated with symptoms of sciatica and herpes, among others.

To a 5-ml, colored-glass, euro-dropper bottle add:

Cypress: 20 drops

Sweet Marjoram: 20 drops

Lavender: 15 drops

Ylang Ylang III: 20 drops

German Chamomile: 20 drops

Black Pepper: 5 drops

Close the cap tightly and shake the bottle vigorously to thoroughly blend the essential oils. Allow to synergize for 8 or more hours before using.

Add 15–18 drops of your synergy blend to a 1-ounce (30-ml) bottle of your favorite carrier oil. Shake the bottle well to disperse the oils thoroughly. Apply a few drops and massage in to relieve nerve pain. Taking a hot shower or bath before applying will increase blood flow to enhance your results. Applying just before bed can be helpful for promoting deep and restful sleep, as well as supporting deep healing and recovery. It may also be effective as a hot compress.

Sciatica Pain Relief Formula

The word *sciatica* dates back to 1451. It is a medical condition characterized by shooting pain that usually radiates down one leg from the lower back. There may also be associated weakness or numbness present in the leg and foot. It's estimated that up to 40 percent of all people will have sciatica at some time in their life.

To a 5-ml, colored-glass, euro-dropper bottle add:

Cypress: 10 drops

Sweet Marjoram: 20 drops

Ylang Ylang III: 20 drops

German Chamomile: 40 drops

Black Pepper: 10 drops

Close the cap tightly and shake the bottle vigorously to thoroughly blend the essential oils. Allow to synergize for 8 or more hours before using.

Add 15–18 drops of your synergy blend to a 1-ounce (30-ml) bottle of your favorite carrier oil. Shake the bottle well to disperse the oils thoroughly. Apply a few drops and massage in to relieve sciatica pain. Taking a hot shower or bath before applying will increase blood flow to enhance your results. Applying just before bed can be helpful for promoting deep and restful sleep, as well as supporting deep healing and recovery. It may also be effective as a hot compress.

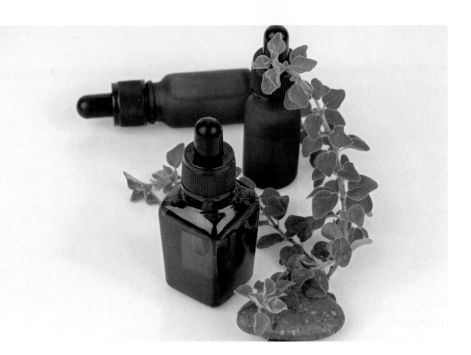

Fibromyalgia Pain Relief Formula

Recognized as a disorder by the U.S. National Institutes of Health and the American College of Rheumatology, fibromyalgia is a chronic, widespread and painful medical condition of the muscles and surrounding connective tissues characterized by an increased response to pressure from the outside environment. Fibromyalgia seems genetically inherited through the family of origin and is often associated with chronic fatigue. Other associated symptoms include anxiety and depression, poor digestion, bowel and bladder issues, post-traumatic stress disorder and sensitivity to light, sound and temperature.

Natural treatment of fibromyalgia includes getting plenty of rest, exercising regularly and eating a whole-foods diet. Essential oils can play an important role as a comfort care measure to alleviate the painful symptoms associated with fibromyalgia.

To a 5-ml, colored-glass, euro-dropper bottle add:
Cypress: 20 drops
Sweet Marjoram: 30 drops
Ylang Ylang III: 30 drops
Peppermint: 20 drops

Close the cap tightly and shake the bottle vigorously to thoroughly blend the essential oils. Allow to synergize for 8 or more hours before using.

Add 15–18 drops of your synergy blend to a 1-ounce (30-ml) bottle of your favorite carrier oil. Shake the bottle well to disperse the oils thoroughly. Apply a few drops and massage in to relieve fibromyalgia or rheumatic pain. Taking a hot shower or bath before applying will increase blood flow to enhance your results. Applying just before bed can be helpful for promoting deep and restful sleep, as well as supporting deep healing and recovery. It may also be effective as a hot compress.

Arthritis Pain Relief Formula

Arthritis is a joint disorder characterized by chronic pain, inflammation and swelling of one or more joints. There are many kinds of arthritis with the most common being osteoarthritis. Getting adequate rest and eating a healthy, whole-foods diet can be helpful. Studies show that regular exercise helps increase range of motion and flexibility and strengthens the joints and the entire physical body.

To a 5-ml, colored-glass, euro-dropper bottle add:

Cypress: 20 drops

Sweet Marjoram: 20 drops

Ylang Ylang III: 20 drops

Peppermint: 20 drops

Black Pepper: 10 drops

Ginger: 10 drops

Close the cap tightly and shake the bottle vigorously to thoroughly blend the essential oils. Allow to synergize for 8 or more hours before using.

Add 15–18 drops of your synergy blend to a 1-ounce (30-ml) bottle of your favorite carrier oil. Shake the bottle well to disperse the oils thoroughly. Apply a few drops and massage in to relieve arthritic-type pain. Taking a hot shower or bath before applying will increase blood flow to enhance your results. Applying just before bed can be helpful for promoting deep and restful sleep, as well as supporting deep healing and recovery. It may also be effective as a hot compress.

Tendinitis Relief Formula

Tendinitis is characterized by pain and inflammation of a tendon and is most commonly caused by excessive overuse or strain. Most commonly, tendinitis injuries occur in the upper shoulder girdle and rotator cuff attachments, as well as the elbow region; however, injury to the Achilles tendon is also quite common.

From years of treating tendinitis injuries, I've learned that the best methods of treatment include complete rest from using the injured tendon for a period of time—up to 6 weeks—along with hot and cold contrasting aromatherapy baths, ice packs and hot compresses. Otherwise, tendinitis can develop into its chronic cousin tendinosis, which is much more challenging to treat and requires a different treatment protocol.

To a 5-ml, colored-glass, euro-dropper bottle add:

Sweet Marjoram: 40 drops

German Chamomile: 20 drops

Helichrysum: 20 drops

Black Pepper: 10 drops

Ginger: 10 drops

Close the cap tightly and shake the bottle vigorously to thoroughly blend the essential oils. Allow to synergize for 8 or more hours before using.

If you're using a 10 percent dilution of any of the pure essential oils, add them directly to your bottle of carrier oil before application.

To make a topical, ready-to-use oil, simply add 18 drops of your formula to a plastic dispensing bottle filled with your chosen carrier oil. Shake well to disperse the oils in the carrier before applying 1–3 drops and massaging into the area. This formula may also be effective as a contrasting hot and cold aromatherapy bath or compress.

Leg Cramp Relief Formula

Leg cramps can be extremely painful and occur suddenly without notice as a usually voluntary leg muscle or muscle group suddenly goes into an excessive involuntary contraction, causing extreme shortening of the leg muscle tissue. A leg cramp can last for several seconds, minutes or even hours. Though the associated cause is not completely understood, cramping of a skeletal muscle, such as leg cramps, may be from excessive exercise, dehydration, low levels of minerals (magnesium, potassium, calcium and sodium) or poor circulation.

It's reported that "around 40% of people who experience skeletal cramps are likely to endure extreme muscle pain, and may be unable to use the entire limb that contains the 'locked-up' muscle group. It may take up to seven days for the muscle to return to a pain-free state."

Leg cramps may occur anytime; however, a large number of them are nocturnal, which means they happen at night, disrupting your normal sleep.

To a 5-ml, colored-glass, euro-dropper bottle add:

Sweet Marjoram: 40 drops

Peppermint: 20 drops

Cypress: 20 drops

Lavender: 10 drops

Helichrysum: 10 drops

Close the cap tightly and shake the bottle vigorously to thoroughly blend the essential oils. Allow to synergize for 8 or more hours before using.

If you're using a 10 percent dilution of any of the pure essential oils, add them directly to your carrier oil.

To make a ready-to-use oil, simply add 10–15 drops of your formula to a plastic dispensing bottle filled with your chosen carrier oil. Shake well to disperse the oils in the carrier before applying gently to the area of leg cramping. Clients report that applying the Leg Cramp Relief Formula after taking a warm shower or bath and just before bed helps them sleep more deeply and prevents nocturnal leg cramps.

Constipation Relief Formula

Constipation has been linked to many illnesses and health risks, including vitamin and mineral deficiency, poor immune response, toxicity, poisoning and a variety of chronic pain syndromes and food allergies.

The Constipation Relief Formula has a distinctly rejuvenating and warming effect and contains essential oils with calming, astringent and restorative properties known to be effective for stimulating digestion and assimilation and for promoting healthy functioning of the stomach, pancreas and intestines.

To a 5-ml, colored-glass, euro-dropper bottle add:
Basil: 10 drops
Cypress: 20 drops
Sweet Orange: 20 drops
Sweet Marjoram: 20 drops
Black Pepper: 10 drops
Peppermint: 20 drops

Close the cap tightly and shake the bottle vigorously to thoroughly blend the essential oils. Allow to synergize for 8 or more hours before using.

Use 10–15 drops of your Constipation Relief Formula on a poultice as a hot compress over the lower abdomen or in a sitz bath (page 95) to promote relief of constipation symptoms. You may repeat as needed.

Nausea Relief Formula

Nausea is an unsettled sensation in your upper stomach that causes you to feel sick. Feelings of nausea can trigger an involuntary urge to vomit and hinder daily activity. Common causes associated with nausea include motion sickness, vertigo, dizziness, migraine, stomach flu, depression, anxiety, medications and food poisoning.

To a 5-ml, colored-glass, euro-dropper bottle add:
Peppermint: 60 drops
Ginger: 20 drops
Lemon: 20 drops

Cap the bottle tightly and shake vigorously to blend the essential oils. Allow to synergize for 8 hours or longer before using.

Dispense 1–3 drops on a cotton ball or smell strip and inhale the aromatic vapors of your Nausea Relief Formula for 10–15 seconds. You may repeat as needed. This formula is also effective when diffused into the air.

To make a ready-to-use nausea relief blend, simply add 15–30 drops of your synergy blend to a 1-ounce (30-ml) bottle of your favorite carrier oil. Shake the bottle well to disperse the oils thoroughly. Apply a few drops of your ready-to-use nausea relief blend to sinus points around your nose and forehead, as well as on the back of your neck.

CAUTION: Though research shows ginger and peppermint to be effective for nausea relief, pregnant women should not use without supervision of a qualified health professional or aromatherapist due to their stimulating effect.

Burn Care Formula

Burns can be caused by heat, radiation, electricity or friction, though statistics show most result from fires and hot liquids. Substance abuse and smoking have also been linked to the probability of getting burns.

There are four kinds of burns. First-degree burns affect the superficial layers of the skin. These are red without blisters, result in minimal pain and last only a few days. Next, there are second-degree burns that cover a larger area of skin with blistering and more intense pain. These require more time to heal and may result in scarring. A third-degree burn covers an even larger area and often has no pain due to nerve damage, and the area is stiff. This type of burn requires special treatment for healing to occur, as the tissue is so injured the body's own natural healing ability needs assistance. A fourth-degree burn involves an even larger area of tissue and may include muscles, tendons or bones, which may be charred black. This can lead to the loss of the injured body part.

The essential oils in this formula have been shown to be effective as a comfort care measure for relieving painful symptoms associated with first- and second-degree burns, as well as for stimulating the body's own natural healing ability to promote rapid healing and prevent scarring.

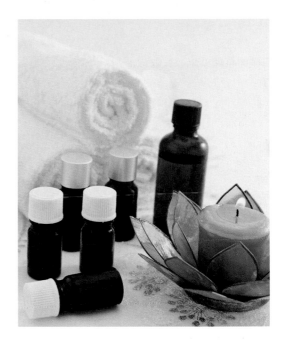

To a 5-ml, colored-glass, euro-dropper bottle add:

German Chamomile: 20 drops

Lavender: 40 drops

Helichrysum: 20 drops

Geranium Roseum and Graveolens: 10 drops each

Close the cap tightly and shake the bottle vigorously to thoroughly blend the essential oils. Allow to synergize for 8 or more hours before using.

If you're using a 10 percent dilution of any of the pure essential oils, add them directly to your carrier oil.

Add 10–15 drops of your pure essential oil Burn Care Formula to a 1-ounce (30-ml) colored-glass misting bottle. Shake the bottle well each time before using to disperse the oils in the water. Gently mist around the burn area to promote fast cooling relief and healing of the tissue.

To make a burn care gel or oil, simply add 10–15 drops of your formula to a plastic dispensing bottle filled with your chosen carrier of aloe vera gel or oil. Shake well to disperse the oils in the carrier before applying gently around the burn area. This formula may also be effective as a cool compress. Clients report it has prevented peeling and scarring of tissue.

Sunburn Relief Formula

Sunburn results from an overexposure to ultra-violet light, most often from the sun. Symptoms of overexposure include reddening of skin tissue that feels hot and painful to the touch; light-headedness or low energy may also result. As the skin heals, it may peel as new skin tissue is formed and, in extreme cases, overexposure may result in permanent scarring of skin tissue. Excess exposure to the sun's ultraviolet light is also the primary cause of non-malignant skin tumors.

As a preventative measure, sun protection such as hats and long sleeves are advised when in the sun for long periods or during the peak hours of midday sun. Sunscreen is another way to prevent sunburn. It has been shown that moderate exposure to the sun that results in sun tanning can actually prevent sunburn as it increases the melanin content in your skin, which is the skin's natural protection against overexposure to the sun.

The essential oils in this formula have been shown effective as a comfort care measure for relieving painful symptoms of sunburn, as well as stimulating your body's own natural healing response, and it may prevent peeling.

To a 5-ml, colored-glass, euro-dropper bottle add:

German Chamomile: 20 drops

Blue Tansy: 20 drops

Lavender: 30 drops

Helichrysum: 20 drops

Rose: 10 drops

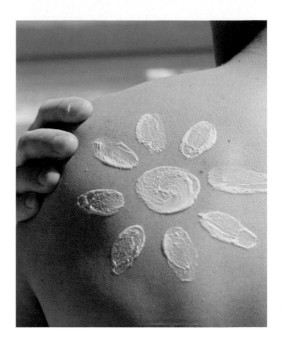

Close the cap tightly and shake the bottle vigorously to thoroughly blend the essential oils. Allow to synergize for 8 or more hours before using.

If you're using a 10-percent dilution of any of the pure essential oils, add them directly to your carrier oil.

Add 10–15 drops of your Sunburn Relief Formula to a 1-ounce (30-ml) colored-glass misting bottle. Shake the bottle well each time before using to disperse the oils in the water. Gently mist around the burn area to promote fast cooling relief and healing of the tissue.

To make a sunburn care gel or oil, simply add 10–15 drops of your formula to a plastic dispensing bottle filled with your chosen carrier of aloe vera gel or oil. Shake well to disperse the oils in the carrier before applying gently around the burned area. This formula may also be effective as a cool compress. Clients report it has prevented peeling and scarring of tissue.

UV Radiation Burn Relief Formula

Damage to the skin may occur with excessive UV radiation that results in redness, inflammation and swelling to the damaged skin and surrounding area. The sun is the most common cause of high exposure to ultraviolet light, but radiation therapy when undergoing cancer treatment is another cause of radiation burns. The oils in this formula have been shown to be effective for relieving the painful symptoms associated with radiation burns, as well as helpful for stimulating natural healing of tissue with little or no peeling of tissue or scarring afterward.

To a 5-ml, colored-glass, euro-dropper bottle add:

German Chamomile: 20 drops

Blue Tansy: 40 drops

Geranium Roseum and Graveolens: 10 drops each

Lavender: 10 drops

Helichrysum: 10 drops

Close the cap tightly and shake the bottle vigorously to thoroughly blend the essential oils. Allow to synergize for 8 or more hours before using.

If you're using a 10 percent dilution of any of the pure essential oils, add them directly to your carrier oil.

Add 10–15 drops of your pure essential oil burn care formula to a 1-ounce (30-ml) colored-glass misting bottle. Shake the bottle well each time before using to disperse the oils in the water. Gently mist around the burn area to promote fast cooling relief and healing of the tissue.

To make a burn care gel or oil, simply add 10–15 drops of your formula to a plastic dispensing bottle filled with your chosen carrier of aloe vera gel or oil. Shake well to disperse the oils in the carrier before applying gently around the burn area. This formula may also be effective as a cool compress. Clients report it has prevented peeling and scarring of tissue.

Mosquito and Insect Protective Repellent Formula

Generally regarded as pests, both mosquitoes and insects are usually very small in size, but can be a huge nuisance or even dangerous to one's health. The mosquito itself feeds on the blood of its hosts, and its saliva can cause irritation to the skin with uncomfortable symptoms like burning and itching. Some mosquitoes are known to pass on very harmful and serious infections like malaria, West Nile virus and dengue fever.

All of the essential oils in this formula are known to protect against mosquito and insect bites, some of which can be quite serious. Research studies have actually shown that peppermint oil not only repels insects in general, but the dengue-fever carrying mosquito as well.

To a 5-ml, colored-glass, euro-dropper bottle add:

Palmarosa: 40 drops

Lemongrass: 20 drops

Lemon Tea Tree: 10 drops

Atlas Cedarwood: 10 drops

Patchouli: 10 drops

Peppermint: 10 drops

Close the cap tightly and shake the bottle vigorously to thoroughly blend the essential oils. Allow to synergize for 8 or more hours before using.

If you're using a 10 percent dilution of any of the pure essential oils, add them directly to your carrier oil.

(continued)

Add 10–15 drops of your pure essential oil formula to a 1-ounce (30-ml) colored-glass misting bottle filled with either purified water or light coconut oil. Light coconut oil has a light enough consistency that it will not clog the atomizer sprayer. Shake the bottle well each time before using to disperse the oils. Gently mist onto clothing or around an area you wish to protect from mosquito and insect bites. You will only need to shake the bottle with carrier oil vigorously once to disperse the oils evenly before using. The oil will stay on longer and have a longer lasting effect. You can also dispense drops of pure essential oil formula on a pool of melted candle wax or in an aroma lamp to diffuse into the air.

Poison Ivy and Oak Irritation Relief Formula

More than 50 million people annually are affected by allergic reactions to poison ivy and poison oak. Only a small percentage of people, about 15–30 percent, have no allergic reaction.

Poison ivy and oak have similar symptoms for which essential oils can be used as a natural remedy to control symptoms and speed healing. Symptoms include burning, itching, reddish inflammation, swelling, irritating skin lesions, non-colored bumps, painful rash and oozing blisters.

Poison ivy and oak aren't spread by touching the blisters themselves, but rather by having direct contact with the oily fluid inside the blisters that can stay on your skin and clothes. That's why it's important for you to wash your hands and all clothing soon after exposure.

To a 5-ml, colored-glass, euro-dropper bottle add:
German Chamomile: 20 drops
Blue Tansy: 20 drops
Helichrysum: 20 drops
Palmarosa: 20 drops
Blue Yarrow: 10 drops
Cypress: 10 drops

Close the cap tightly and shake the bottle vigorously to thoroughly blend the essential oils. Allow to synergize for 8 or more hours before using.

If you're using a 10 percent dilution of any of the pure essential oils, add them directly to your carrier oil.

Add 10–15 drops of your pure essential oil Poison Ivy and Oak Irritation Relief Formula to a 1-ounce (30-ml) colored-glass misting bottle filled with purified water. Shake the bottle well each time before using to disperse the oils in the water. Mist around the affected area to promote fast relief of symptoms and speed healing.

To make a leave-on gel or oil, simply add 10–15 drops of your formula to a plastic dispensing bottle filled with your chosen carrier of aloe vera gel or oil. Shake well to disperse the oils in the carrier before applying gently around the area. This formula may also be effective as a cool compress or in a bath. Be sure to wash hands thoroughly with a sanitizing agent after direct contact with poison oak or ivy on the skin.

Allergic Skin Reaction Relief Formula

Allergic skin reactions are a hypersensitive immune response to a substance that triggers abnormal symptoms like itching, burning, blisters, redness, rash, pain, hives, swelling and inflammation.

Allergies are common. Reports indicate that about 20 percent of people have experienced a skin reaction like eczema, which is common among young children.

There are many substances that can trigger an allergic skin reaction, including:

- Insect bites from bees, wasps and spiders
- Common foods (i.e., gluten, eggs, dairy, nuts and fruits)
- Chemicals or medications
- Metals (i.e., gold in jewelry)

The best way to avoid allergic skin reactions is to eliminate the allergens that cause them.

To a 5-ml, colored-glass, euro-dropper bottle add:

Blue Yarrow: 20 drops

Ylang Ylang III: 20 drops

Palmarosa: 30 drops

Geranium Roseum and Graveolens: 5 drops each

German Chamomile: 10 drops

Helichrysum: 10 drops

Close the cap tightly and shake the bottle vigorously to thoroughly blend the essential oils. Allow to synergize for 8 or more hours before using.

If you're using a 10 percent dilution of any of the pure essential oils, add them directly to your carrier before application.

Dispense 1–3 drops on a cotton ball or smell strip and inhale the aromatic vapors of your blend for 10–15 seconds to promote calming of your immune system and allergic response. You may repeat as needed.

Add 10–15 drops of your pure essential oil Allergic Skin Reaction Relief Formula to a 1-ounce (30-ml) colored-glass misting bottle. Shake the bottle well each time before using to disperse the oils in the water. Mist gently around the area of the allergic skin reaction.

To make a topical gel or oil, simply add 10–15 drops of your formula to a plastic dispensing bottle filled with your chosen carrier of aloe vera gel or oil (light coconut oil recommended). Shake well to disperse the oils in the carrier before applying gently around the affected area. Avoid direct application onto the allergic skin reaction until the skin has begun to clear. This formula may also be effective as a cool compress.

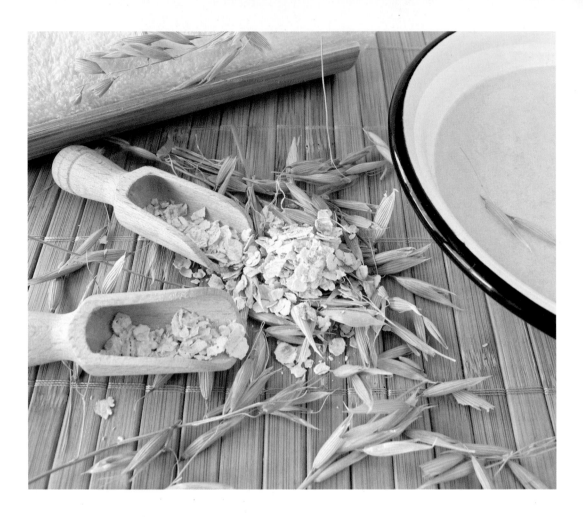

Warm Bath Treatment

A warm bath can bring relief when nothing else will. Especially good for soothing allergic skin reactions, baths may also be used to relieve poison ivy and oak irritations.

Allergic Skin Reaction Relief Formula (page 69)

4 cups (90 g) raw, uncooked oats

In a bowl, add 10–15 drops of your essential oil blend to 4 cups (90 g) of raw, uncooked oats. Mix the blend thoroughly into the oats, cover and set aside while you draw a warm bath. Add the oats with the essential oil blend to your bath water and stir into the water. Relax in the bath for 10–20 minutes. This method of treatment is especially good for soothing an outbreak of hives.

CAUTION: You may wish to do a skin allergy test for each of the essential oils in the formula before using.

Scar Formula

Scars naturally occur on areas of the skin after there has been an injury. Scar tissue formation, which is made up of protein (collagen), is a normal function of tissue repair after an injury, and the appearance of scarring is common.

A scar treatment of essential oils is most effective when applied immediately after an injury to the skin, though even old scars can become noticeably less apparent or even disappear completely. This depends upon the severity of the injury to the skin, the age of the scar and other factors like diet and quality of skin tissue.

To a 5-ml, colored-glass, euro-dropper bottle add:

Helichrysum: 20 drops

German Chamomile: 20 drops

Rose: 20 drops

Palmarosa: 10 drops

Geranium Roseum and Graveolens: 5 drops each

Ylang Ylang: 5 drops

Carrot Seed: 5 drops

Lavender: 5 drops

Myrrh: 5 drops

Close the cap tightly and shake the bottle vigorously to thoroughly blend the essential oils. Allow to synergize for 8 or more hours before using.

If you're using a 10 percent dilution of any of the pure essential oils, add them directly to your carrier oil and shake well to blend before application to the skin.

To make a ready-to-use dilution for direct application to the skin, add 10–15 drops of your pure essential oil Scar Formula to a 1-ounce (30-ml) plastic dispensing bottle. Or you can add 5–8 drops of formula to a 0.5-ounce (15-ml) colored-glass, euro-dropper bottle filled with your chosen carrier oil. Shake well to disperse the oils in the carrier before gently applying to the area of the scar. This may be applied first as a warm compress (to soften tissue) before applying the ready-to-use blend.

Athlete's Foot Formula

Athlete's foot is a common infection of the feet caused by a fungus. The medical term used for it is *tinea pedis*. Some of the characteristic signs and symptoms associated with athlete's foot are redness, itching, burning, peeling and blisters. As fungal infections thrive in moist environments, between the toes of the feet are the most commonly infected areas because of poor air circulation to keep the area dry. Fungal infections may also occur on the hands and toenails, as well as the fingernails.

To a 5-ml, colored-glass, euro-dropper bottle add:

Clove: 40 drops

Tea Tree: 20 drops

Thyme: 20 drops

Lemon: 20 drops

¼ cup (130 g) Epsom or sea salts

Foot bath

(continued)

Close the cap tightly and shake the bottle vigorously to thoroughly blend the essential oils. Allow to synergize for 8 or more hours before using.

Add 10–15 drops of your pure essential oil Athlete's Foot Formula to a carrier of ¼ cup (130 g) Epsom or sea salts and mix thoroughly. You can add more drops of the athlete's foot blend in subsequent foot baths if well tolerated.

Fill your foot bath with hot water (98°F–101°F [37°C–38°C]), add scented salts and stir into foot bath water completely. Soak your foot/feet for 15–20 minutes or until the water cools. Dry with a clean hand towel.

Next, apply a 10 percent, ready-to-use dilution of the athlete's foot fungus blend around the infection to be absorbed into your skin.

It's best to leave your feet open to the air and keep the area as dry as possible; wearing open sandals may be helpful. You may apply your ready-to-use blend as often as needed between foot soaks. Be sure to wash your hands thoroughly with a sanitizing cleanser after direct contact with the infected area.

Perform your athlete's foot bath at least once or twice daily for 3–6 weeks, or even longer in some cases, depending upon how severe your case of athlete's foot is.

Toenail Fungus Formula

The medical term for toenail fungus is *tinea unguium*. Though it may also affect the fingernails, the most common malady of the nail is toenail fungus, which affects 10 percent of the population.

Toenail fungus appears as a thickened, brittle and discolored nail bed varying in colors from a black, reddish orange to yellow and green. As the infection worsens, the nail begins to break down and pieces of the nail detach from the nail bed, which becomes red, inflamed and painful. Advanced toenail fungus can also have quite an offensive smell.

Research shows that the most important factors for preventing a toenail fungal infection are good blood circulation and ventilation of the toes and feet. Also, toenail fungus seems to run in the family, so if your father had toenail fungus you're far more likely to have it yourself. Men are far more often affected by the disease than women.

Essential oils are effective for destroying a toenail fungal infection, promoting healing of the nail bed and stimulating growth of a new nail matrix.

To a 5-ml, colored-glass, euro-dropper bottle add:
Clove Bud: 30 drops

Myrrh: 30 drops

Lemon: 20 drops

Thyme: 10 drops

Lavender: 10 drops

¼ cup (130 g) Epsom or sea salts
Foot bath

Close the cap tightly and shake the bottle vigorously to thoroughly blend the essential oils. Allow to synergize for 8 or more hours before using.

Add 10–15 drops of your pure essential oil Toenail Fungus Formula to a carrier of ¼ cup (130 g) Epsom or sea salts and mix thoroughly. You can add more drops of the toenail fungus blend in subsequent foot baths if well tolerated.

Fill your foot bath with hot water (98°F–101°F [37°C–38°C]), add scented salts and stir into foot bath water completely. Soak your foot/feet for 15–20 minutes or until the water cools. Dry with a clean hand towel.

Next, apply a 10 percent, ready-to-use dilution of the toenail fungus blend around the infection to be absorbed into your skin.

It's best to leave your feet open to the air and keep the area as dry as possible; wearing open sandals may be helpful. You may apply your ready-to-use blend as often as needed between foot soaks. Be sure to wash your hands thoroughly with a sanitizing cleanser after direct contact with the infected area. Perform your toenail fungus footbath at least once or twice daily for 3–6 weeks, or even longer in some cases, depending upon how severe your case of toenail fungus is.

Foot Bath for Athlete's Foot or Toenail Fungus

A foot bath is a way to focus your essential oils to a specific area. The warm water increases circulation and action of oils.

---

1 cup (500 g) Epsom or sea salts

10–15 drops Athlete's Foot Formula (page 71) or Toenail Fungus Formula (page 72)

Foot bath

In small ceramic bowl, combine 1 cup (500 g) salts and 10–15 drops of the essential oils formula. Blend in thoroughly and set aside. Fill your foot bath with hot water (98°F–101°F [37°C–38°C]). Add the scented salts into the foot bath water and stir. Soak your foot/feet, being sure to submerge and cover the toenails completely in water. Soak for 10–20 minutes or until the water cools. Towel dry and allow the area to remain open to the air as much as possible. Wearing open-toed sandals can be helpful.

For Use in Between Foot Baths

Add 10–15 drops of your pure essential oil formula to a 1-ounce (30-ml) colored-glass misting bottle filled with light coconut oil. Light coconut oil will not clog the atomizer sprayer. Shake the bottle vigorously to disperse the oils before applying to the affected area.

To make a gel or oil, simply add 10–15 drops of your formula to a plastic dispensing bottle filled with your chosen carrier of aloe vera gel or oil. Shake well to disperse the oils in the carrier before applying. Be sure to wash hands thoroughly with a sanitizing agent after direct contact with the area.

Warts Formula (Non-genital)

Warts are usually small, rough patches of growth that look somewhat like a head of cauliflower. They are caused by a viral infection, and common areas of infection are the hands and feet. Though the common wart is considered benign, its appearance causes concern for many, especially children and young adults, with a 12–24 percent rate of occurrence. Warts are contagious and may spread through contact with open areas and broken skin.

To a 5-ml, colored-glass, euro-dropper bottle add:

Tea Tree: 10 drops

Cinnamon Leaf: 20 drops

Lemon: 20 drops

Thyme: 10 drops

Myrrh: 20 drops

Clove Bud: 20 drops

¼ cup (130 g) Epsom or sea salts

Foot bath

Close the cap tightly and shake the bottle vigorously to thoroughly blend the essential oils. Allow to synergize for 8 or more hours before using.

Add 10–15 drops of your pure essential oil Wart Formula to a carrier of ¼ cup (130 g) of Epsom or sea salts and mix thoroughly. You can add more drops of the wart blend in subsequent footbaths if well tolerated.

Fill your footbath with hot water (98°F–101°F [37°C–38°C]), add scented salts and stir into the foot bath water completely. Soak the area of your wart for 15–20 minutes or until the water cools. Dry with a clean hand towel.

Next, apply a 10 percent, ready-to-use dilution of the wart blend directly on the wart, and let the oils be absorbed into the skin.

It's best to leave the wart open to the air and keep the area as dry as possible. You may apply your ready-to-use wart blend as often as needed between soaks. Be sure to wash your hands thoroughly with a sanitizing cleanser after direct contact with the infected area.

Perform your wart bath at least once or twice daily for 3–6 weeks or even longer in some cases.

Herpes Formula

There are two types of herpes simplex virus, type 1 (HSV-1) and type 2 (HSV-2). Herpes simplex-1 is more common, affects the mouth and is referred to as a cold sore. HSV-2 is what causes the genital type of herpes infections. Both are transmittable by direct contact with the body fluids and lesions of an infected individual. The communicable disease may still be transmitted even when asymptomatic. Genital herpes is considered a sexually transmitted disease (STD). Though condom use can decrease the risk of infection, the most effective prevention is to avoid any genital contact. At the start of this millennium, it was estimated that more than 536 million people (16 percent of the world's population) were infected with HSV-2. Most people with HSV-2 are asymptomatic and do not realize that they are infected.

This formula contains some of the most potent antimicrobial and antiviral essential oils known in aromatherapy and may be helpful for promoting relief and faster healing for symptoms of herpes outbreaks. Be careful to apply the herpes formula around the herpes lesion, not directly on an open lesion!

To a 5-ml, colored-glass, euro-dropper bottle add:

Bergamot: 20 drops

Palmarosa: 20 drops

Myrrh: 10 drops

Helichrysum: 10 drops

Rose: 10 drops

Cypress: 5 drops

Lavender: 5 drops

Lemon: 5 drops

Oregano: 1 drop

Thyme: 1 drop

Galbanum: 5 drops

Close the cap tightly and shake the bottle vigorously to thoroughly blend the essential oils. Allow to synergize for 8 or more hours before using.

If you're using a 10 percent dilution of any of the pure essential oils, add them directly to your carrier oil.

Add 10–15 drops of your pure essential oil formula to a 1-ounce (30-ml) colored-glass misting bottle of purified water or light coconut oil. Light coconut oil is light enough that it will not clog your atomizer sprayer. Shake the bottle well each time before using to disperse the oils in the water. Lightly mist around the area of the herpes outbreak to promote fast relief and healing of tissue. If using light coconut oil, you will only need to shake the bottle vigorously once to disperse the oils evenly in the carrier before using.

To make a herpes ready-to-use gel, simply add 10–15 drops of your formula to a plastic dispensing bottle filled with your chosen carrier of aloe vera gel. Shake well to disperse the oils in the carrier before applying gently around the infected area. This formula may also be effective as a cool or warm compress.

CAUTION: Oregano oil is a potent, "hot" antimicrobial and should be used with extreme caution. As it is a strong irritant to the skin and mucous membranes, use a less than 1 percent dilution for safe skin application. Avoid during pregnancy and with young children and pets.

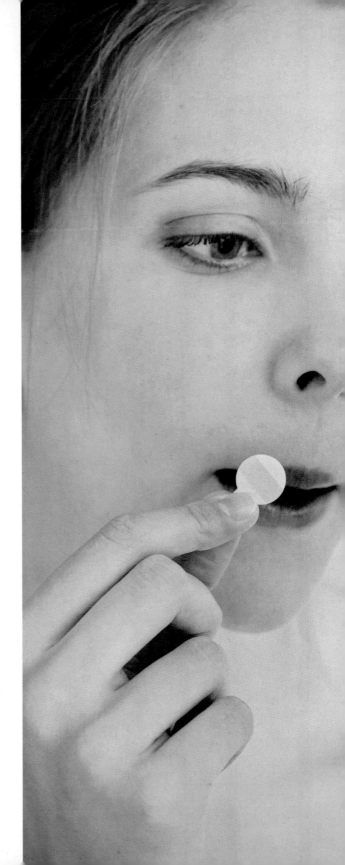

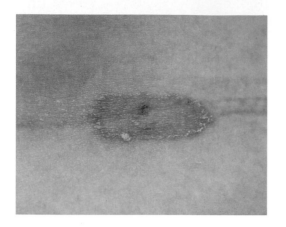

Ringworm Formula

Ringworm is caused by a fungal infection of the skin. The medical term for ringworm is *dermatophytosis*. As with all fungi, ringworm thrives in warm, moist environments where there is little or no air circulation. It's thought that 20 percent or more of the population is infected with ringworm, with athletes being the most commonly affected by this skin condition.

Ringworm appears as enlarged raised rings of the fungi on the skin and thus the name ringworm. An infection on the skin of the feet by dermatophytosis is called athlete's foot and in the groin it is called jock itch. Ringworm is contagious and spreads between humans. Animals, including dogs and cats, can also become infected by the disease.

Signs of ringworm infection include:

- Raised red, itchy patches on the skin that resemble a ring
- Red patches with blisters that drain and ooze
- Bald patches on the scalp or fur of an animal
- Discoloration and cracking in severe cases

Fungi like ringworm thrive in warm, moist environments and are often picked up in public shared facilities like gyms, saunas or swimming pools. Sharing exercise equipment that has not been disinfected properly and communal sharing of towels and other wearable gear is considered to be the primary cause of the disease. The number one prevention method is to avoid sharing clothing and sports equipment and to always wear protective footwear like thongs when using public facilities.

To a 5-ml, colored-glass, euro-dropper bottle add:
German Chamomile: 20 drops
Blue Tansy: 20 drops
Palmarosa: 20 drops
Spikenard: 20 drops
Helichrysum: 10 drops
Lavender: 10 drops

Close the cap tightly and shake the bottle vigorously to thoroughly blend the essential oils. Allow to synergize for 8 or more hours before using.

If you're using a 10 percent dilution of any of the pure essential oils, add them directly to your carrier oil.

Add 10–15 drops of your pure essential oil Ringworm Formula to a 1-ounce (30-ml) colored-glass misting bottle filled with purified water. Shake the bottle well each time before using to disperse the oils in the water. Lightly mist around the area to promote fast relief of itching and to promote healing.

To make a ringworm gel or oil, simply add 10–15 drops of your formula to a plastic dispensing bottle filled with your chosen carrier of aloe vera gel or oil. Shake well to disperse the oils in the carrier before applying gently around the area. This formula may also be effective as a cool compress. Always thoroughly wash your hands with a sanitizing soap after direct contact with the infection.

Ringing Ear Relief Formula

The medical term for ringing ear is *tinnitus,* which comes from the Latin word *tinnīre* meaning "to ring." Tinnitus is often described as a ringing or buzzing sound, though sometimes clicking, roaring and hissing are other terms used to describe the sound. It can come from one or both ears and be either loud or soft and high or low pitched. Ringing ear can cause depression, nervousness and anxiety in 1–2 percent of people, while most tolerate it very well. Tinnitus is thought to be brought on from a number of causes such as ear infections, stress, certain medications, allergies, Ménière's disease, head injury, nerve damage, poor circulation or earwax buildup.

Preventative care includes avoiding listening to loud music, especially through headphones.

The Ringing Ear Relief Formula contains essential oils with calming, astringent and restorative properties known to be effective for relieving symptoms of tinnitus, especially when associated with congestion or poor nerve conduction and circulation.

To a 5-ml, colored-glass, euro-dropper bottle add:

Cypress: 20 drops

Lemon: 20 drops

Helichrysum: 40 drops

Birch: 10 drops

Juniper Berry: 10 drops

Close the cap tightly and shake the bottle vigorously to thoroughly blend the essential oils. Allow to synergize for 8 or more hours before using.

Use your Ringing Ear Relief Formula as a poultice to relieve congestion and symptoms related to poor circulation and nerve conduction. You may repeat as needed. To make a ready-to-use Ringing Ear Relief blend, simply add 15–30 drops of your synergy blend to a 1-ounce (30-ml) bottle of your favorite carrier oil. Shake the bottle well to disperse the oils thoroughly. Apply a few drops of your blend to the front and backside of your ear with tinnitus symptoms and massage in.

Sleep Formulas

Studies show that sleep deprivation causes one out of every six fatal car accidents. The research also shows that 17 continuous hours without sleep not only decreases your alertness and performance, but also increases your blood alcohol levels enough for you to be classified as a drunk driver. Disastrous events like the Valdez oil spill and Chernobyl have been linked to human errors due to sleep deprivation.

A modern malady, sleep deprivation was not experienced before the invention of electric lights. Before indoor lighting, people followed their natural sleep cycles, went to bed soon after sunset and rose again at sunrise, which resulted in more hours of sleep.

The research indicates that if it takes you more than 10–15 minutes to fall asleep, then you're sleep deprived. An excellent sign that you are not sleep deprived is when you're tired enough to immediately fall into a deep state of dreamless sleep and wake up feeling refreshed and alert.

The essential oils in both of these sleep formulas promote deep and restful sleep and have been shown effective for relieving symptoms of sleep loss, insomnia and night terrors. They help calm anxiety and worry and are helpful for restoring the body's natural sleep cycles.

Sleep Formula 1

The essential oils in this formula help you relax more easily, so you fall asleep and stay asleep.

To a 5-ml, colored-glass, euro-dropper bottle add:

Lavender: 10 drops

Clary Sage: 10 drops

Ylang Ylang III: 20 drops

German Chamomile: 20 drops

Spikenard: 20 drops

Red Mandarin: 20 drops

Cap the bottle tightly and shake vigorously to blend the essential oils. Allow to synergize for 8 hours or longer before using. If you're using a 10 percent dilution of any of the pure essential oils, add them directly to your bottle of carrier oil before application.

Dispense 1–3 drops on a cotton ball or smell strip and inhale the aromatic vapors of your sleep blend for 10–15 seconds. You may repeat as needed. This formula is also effective when diffused into the air or used as an aromatic spray.

To make a ready-to-use blend, simply add 15–30 drops of your synergy blend to a 1-ounce (30-ml) bottle of your favorite carrier oil. Shake the bottle well to disperse the oils thoroughly. Apply a few drops of your ready-to-use blend to sinus points around your nose and forehead, as well as on the back of your neck. This is also excellent in your bath as a nighttime relaxation soak just before bed.

Sleep Formula 2

This second sleep formula is for those of you who want an alternative sleep formula to try or who wish to avoid the use of clary sage. Some women prefer not to use clary sage, and previously it was thought to have mild phyto (plant) estrogen-like properties.

To a 5-ml, colored-glass, euro-dropper bottle add:

Red Mandarin: 40 drops

Ylang Ylang III: 20 drops

German Chamomile: 20 drops

Spikenard: 10 drops

Vetiver: 10 drops

Cap the bottle tightly and shake vigorously to blend the essential oils. Allow to synergize for 8 hours or longer before using. If you're using a 10 percent dilution of any of the pure essential oils, add them directly to your bottle of carrier oil before application.

Dispense 1–3 drops on a cotton ball or smell strip and inhale the aromatic vapors of your sleep blend for 10–15 seconds. You may repeat as needed. This formula is also effective when diffused into the air or used as an aromatic spray.

To make a ready-to-use blend, simply add 15–30 drops of your synergy blend to a 1-ounce (30-ml) bottle of your favorite carrier oil. Shake the bottle well to disperse the oils thoroughly. Apply a few drops of your ready-to-use blend to sinus points around your nose and forehead, as well as on the back of your neck. This is also excellent in your bath as a nighttime relaxation soak just before bed.

CHAPTER 9

Healthy *Lifestyle*

Cleansing and Detoxification Formula

The body naturally cleanses and detoxifies itself perfectly. Using essential oils for cleansing and detoxification in this context simply means gently stimulating the body's own natural healing processes to enhance cleansing and detoxification. Part of a cleansing and detoxification program might include removing any processed foods and eating only natural whole foods that the body uses more efficiently for cellular regeneration and healing.

A nerve and blood tonic, the detoxification formula contains essential oils with powerful astringent, circulatory and immune stimulant properties. The properties are known to be effective for stimulating lymph drainage and may also be effective for internal cleansing of the liver and gallbladder when abstaining from toxic substances like drugs and alcohol. This blend may also promote heavy metal detoxification (HMD).

To a 5-ml, colored-glass, euro-dropper bottle add:
Juniper Berry: 40 drops
Cypress: 20 drops
Lemon: 20 drops
Myrrh: 10 drops
Rosemary: 10 drops

Close the cap tightly and shake the bottle vigorously to thoroughly blend the essential oils. Allow to synergize for 8 or more hours before using.

Use the Cleansing and Detoxification Formula as a poultice over the liver and gallbladder area or in a bath to promote cleansing and detoxification. You may experiment with other methods of application (refer to the "How to Use Essential Oils" section on page 20) for even more suggestions about how to use the Cleansing and Detoxification Formula to find out what works best for you.

Weight Loss Program

Most people know that dieting doesn't work, and the research shows that the very process of dieting itself increases your body's natural tendency to gain weight. Researchers call this "diet-induced weight gain," and it is considered a factor in the increasing obesity epidemic.

A study of more than 2,000 sets of twins from Finland, from sixteen to twenty-five years of age, showed that after embarking on just one dieting weight loss plan, the dieting twin was two to three times more likely to become overweight compared to the non-dieting twin. Furthermore, with each subsequent restricted plan to lose weight, their risk increased for becoming overweight.

In conclusion, researchers agree, "It is now well established that the more people engage in dieting, the more they gain weight in the long-term."

Restricted food intake or dieting is also associated with food binging, overeating and eating disorders.

Eating Intuitively

For years I've followed my intuition to know what to eat. Over time my intuitive eating style has developed, and I am more fine-tuned to my body's own particular needs for diet and nutrition. I was delighted to find there is research to support what I've known for years about the key to eating right for you as an individual.

Research by Tracy Tylka, PhD, professor of psychology at The Ohio State University, has shown that the healthiest and best way to lose weight naturally is through becoming aware of the needs of your own body and mind. This process of inner-oriented awareness is called "Intuitive Eating." According to the research, dieting interferes with your inner awareness and natural hunger signals that get switched off. By engaging in a program of Intuitive Eating, along with your appetite suppressant, you'll regain awareness and reset your inner guidance system for healthy, natural weight loss.

Key Principles for Eating Intuitively

- Eat when you're hungry and whatever foods you desire.
- Eat for physical nourishment rather than emotional comfort.
- Listen to your internal hunger signals to know when and how much to eat.

Helpful Guidance

1. The first step to healthy, natural weight loss is to be aware that you have a weight-loss issue and dieting doesn't work.

2. Make a firm commitment to healthy natural weight loss. Connect with your motivation and true desire for losing weight. Knowing the reason why you truly desire to lose weight can help you make a firm commitment to changing your belief about yourself as being overweight.

3. Understand why you might be overweight. You probably have psychological and emotional reasons for overeating that operate automatically at the subconscious level. You may believe that eating will give you comfort and help you deal with uncomfortable emotions. Eating can also be like a reward mechanism to get your emotional needs met. Becoming aware of the psychological and emotional rewards that overeating gives you can help you take your power back and disrupt the overeating "habit loop" to break an emotional eating habit.

4. Connect the dots. Becoming aware of the situations that trigger overeating helps you understand what the habit of overeating is giving you as a short-term reward. Becoming aware of the context that triggers your urge to eat helps you break the automatic emotional eating habit. When you feel the urge to eat, take a moment to think about what may have just happened to trigger the urge. Doing so will disrupt the habitual pattern of emotional eating. Write down a few notes about what you're feeling. This helps you to observe your feelings rather than repress them through emotional eating. Observing your uncomfortable feelings helps you to take your power back and to feel more in charge of your situation.

5. Develop a plan of action. Once you become aware and understand what triggers your urge to overeat, make a clear, specific plan of action for how to minimize or even eliminate your habit triggers. It could be that certain environments, people or situations trigger your urge for emotional overeating. Take stock of what supports your new natural weight loss plan and engage in those activities.

6. Be consistent and build momentum. Be the change you wish to see by visualizing yourself at the weight you desire for yourself. Research shows that more than 90 percent of your behavior and habits operate at the unconscious level. Therefore, gaining the support of your subconscious mind through consistent visualization of yourself at your desired weight and seeing yourself in an environment that supports you can be very helpful.

7. Be patient and kind to yourself. Breaking an emotional eating habit can take time. Showing compassion to yourself and being your own best friend through the process has been shown to be helpful for successfully breaking any habit, including emotional eating. Becoming aware of the psychological and emotional triggers that anchor your habit of emotional eating can take time to unravel and disentangle, so be kind and patient with yourself.

Weight Loss Formula and Treatment

Over the past 20 years, obesity has reached epidemic proportions in the United States. According to the National Center for Health Statistics, one-third of the adult population age 20 years and older—over 100 million people—are obese. Children and teenagers are also showing increased rates of obesity. According to research, obesity is now considered primarily a lifestyle issue brought on by poor choice of diet and lack of exercise. The prevalence of obesity is resulting in increased health risks and diseases among adults and children alike. The health risks include:

- High blood pressure (hypertension)
- Heart disease
- Arthritis
- Some cancers (breast, colon, endometrial)
- High cholesterol
- Gallbladder disease
- Stroke

I conducted a small, uncontrolled study of seven women who used a pure essential oil appetite suppressant that I formulated for them. Everyone was instructed not to diet during the use of the appetite suppressant. After 3 weeks all of the women reported weight loss with no dieting or exercise. All but one woman lost between 7–10 pounds (3–5 kg). One woman in the group lost only 1 pound (454 g). What all of the women who lost the 7–10 pounds (3–5 kg) reported was that their awareness about what they were eating significantly changed, and their desire for certain foods naturally lessened or even completely disappeared.

This is the appetite suppressant formula these women used:

To a 5-ml, colored-glass, euro-dropper bottle add:
Lemon: 35 drops
Sweet Orange: 30 drops
Grapefruit: 35 drops
Patchouli: 1 drop

Close the cap tightly and shake the bottle vigorously to thoroughly blend the essential oils. Allow to synergize for 8 or more hours before using.

Dispense 1–3 drops on a cotton ball, a smell strip or a 1-dram, colored-glass vial of Celtic salt (cap tightly and shake to disperse the oils) and inhale the aromatic vapors of your appetite suppressant blend for 10–15 seconds. You may repeat as needed. The formula is also effective diffused into the air.

Weight Loss Formula 2

Essential oils are the pure and natural way to lose weight. You can feel great, enjoy eating the food you love and lose weight when using an appetite suppressant made with essential oils. This weight loss formula has been proven to be effective for suppressing appetite signals that may cause you to eat when you're not hungry, as well as helping you control an excessive sweet tooth.

The oils in this formula are a perfect balance of aromas for curbing your appetite, as well as for increasing your fat burning and metabolism. It will help to relieve food cravings and enhance your digestion. The citrus oils are known to be natural body tonics, to have an alkalizing effect and to promote the cleansing and detoxification that are so important when losing weight. The natural detoxifying oils in this Weight Loss Formula will help free you of some of the uncomfortable side effects of losing weight like headache, fatigue and food cravings.

To a 5-ml, colored-glass, euro-dropper bottle add:

Peppermint: 20 drops

Pink Grapefruit: 30 drops

Lemon: 30 drops

Sweet Orange: 20 drops

Fennel: 1–3 drops

Cap the bottle tightly and shake vigorously to blend the essential oils. Allow to synergize for 8 hours or longer before using.

Dispense 1–3 drops on a cotton ball or smell strip and inhale the aromatic vapors of your Weight Loss Formula 2 for 10–15 seconds. You may repeat as needed. This formula is also effective when diffused into the air.

To make a ready-to-use weight loss blend, simply add 15–30 drops of your synergy blend to a 1-ounce (30-ml) bottle of your favorite carrier oil. Shake the bottle well to disperse the oils thoroughly. Apply a few drops of your ready-to-use weight loss blend to the back of your neck and upper and lower abdomen and massage in thoroughly.

Use your appetite suppressant frequently throughout the day for a minimum of 3 weeks. Inhale the scent of your appetite suppressant before you eat or go food shopping, any time you feel prone to snack or take a second helping and also when you're dining out.

Repetition (and consistency) is the key for getting results. Refer to the "Weight Loss Program" section of this book on page 80 for helpful and supportive information about how to achieve healthy and natural weight loss without dieting.

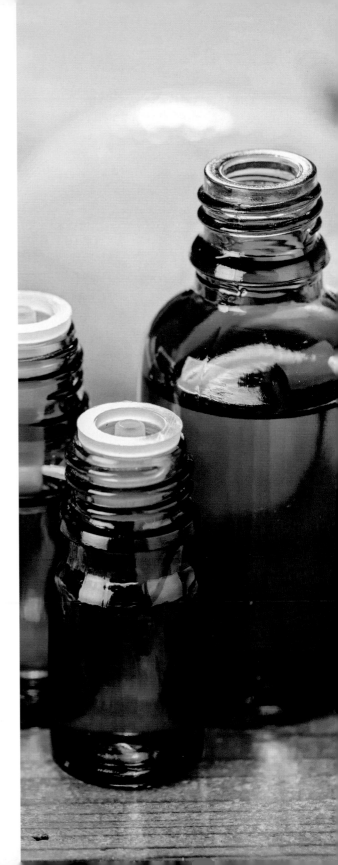

Stop Smoking Program

1. The first step to stopping smoking is to be aware that you have an addiction to smoking and that you want to stop. Some people are able to quit cold turkey, while for others it can take time and effort to break the smoking habit. Research studies show that most people may try numerous times to break the smoking habit before being successful. On a psychological and emotional level, there is an unraveling of your attachments and associations to smoking that anchor your smoking habit primarily in your subconscious mind. You believe yourself to be a smoker, and so you have a smoking habit. To break a smoking habit, you have to create a new image of yourself as a non-smoker, which can take time for some people while others can do it immediately.

2. Make a firm commitment to quit smoking. Connecting your motivation with the reason why you truly desire to quit smoking can help you make a firm decision and commit to changing your belief about yourself as being a non-smoker. Over time, with firm commitment, you build the momentum and follow-through necessary to stop smoking.

3. Understand your smoking habit. You probably have psychological and emotional anchors to your smoking habit that operate automatically. You may believe that smoking helps you relax and deal with uncomfortable emotions, problems and situations in your life. You have an association with smoking as being your friend that you look to for support and comfort when in stressful situations. Smoking can also act like a reward mechanism, and you may believe it helps you accomplish a challenging task. Becoming aware of the psychological and emotional rewards that smoking gives helps you take your power back and disrupt the smoking habit loop.

4. Connect the dots. Becoming aware of the situations that trigger smoking can help you to understand what the habit of smoking is giving you as a short-term reward. Understanding the context that triggers your urge to smoke helps you break the automatic habit. When you feel the urge to smoke, take a moment to become aware of what may have just happened to trigger it. Doing so will disrupt the habitual pattern of smoking. Write down a few notes about what you're feeling. This helps you to observe your feelings rather than repress them by habitually smoking. Observing your uncomfortable feelings helps you to take your power back and to feel more in charge of your situation.

5. Develop a plan of action. Once you become aware of and understand what triggers your urge to smoke, make a clear, specific plan of action for how to minimize or even eliminate your habit triggers. It could be certain environments, people or situations that trigger your urge to smoke. Take stock of what supports your new smoke-free habit and engage in those activities.

6. Be consistent and build momentum. Be the change you wish to see by visualizing yourself as a non-smoker. Visualizing your success has the effect of gaining the cooperation of your subconscious mind to help you to break a smoking habit. Research shows that more than 90 percent of your behavior and habits operate at the unconscious level; therefore, gaining the support of your subconscious mind through consistent visualization of yourself as a non-smoker and seeing yourself in an environment that supports being smoke-free can be very helpful.

7. Breaking a smoking habit can take time. Showing compassion for yourself and being your own best friend through the process has been shown to be helpful for successfully breaking a smoking habit. Becoming aware of the psychological and emotional triggers that anchor your smoking habit can take time to unravel and disentangle, so be kind and patient with yourself.

Research suggests that it takes a minimum of 3 weeks for your established pattern and mental image of yourself to dissolve and a new mental image as a non-smoker to be created, leading to the formation of your new habit.

Other research suggests a minimum of 40 days, while a recent study of ninety-six people published in the *European Journal of Social Psychology* reported that it took an average of 66 days to form a new habit.

With repetition, you build momentum for your new habit to take root in your subconscious. Seeing a picture in your mind of yourself as a non-smoker feels natural and becomes automatic.

Based on this information, you want to use your Stop Smoking Formula continuously for a minimum of 3 weeks and then as needed to maintain your new smoke-free habit.

Stop Smoking Formula and Treatment

Stopping a smoking addiction can be either cold turkey or a long-term plan that involves cutting down smoking over a period of time to eventually quit altogether. Recent psychosocial pressures and the banning of smoking in or near public facilities have resulted in a decrease in the smoking habit. Studies have shown that smoking in the U.S. has continued to decrease since 2005 and has now reached an all-time low, even though the population has increased. Worldwide statistics show that smoking is the leading cause of preventable death. The problem is that nicotine in tobacco is very addictive, and the symptoms of nicotine withdrawal when stopping smoking are very uncomfortable and include anxiety, food cravings, weight gain, agitation and depression.

Essential oils can be helpful not only in helping you to break the nicotine habit, but also in supporting the detoxification process and relieving symptoms of withdrawal.

To a 5-ml, colored-glass, euro-dropper bottle add:
Bergamot: 50 drops
Black Pepper: 40 drops
Rosemary Verbenone: 10 drops

(continued)

Close the cap tightly and shake the bottle vigorously to thoroughly blend the essential oils. Allow to synergize for 8 or more hours before using.

Dispense 1–3 drops of the Stop Smoking Formula blend onto a cotton ball or smell strip and inhale the aromatic vapors for 10–15 seconds. This formula is also effective in a diffuser or as an aromatic mist. To make a ready-to-use stop smoking blend, simply add 15–30 drops of your synergy blend to a 1-ounce (30-ml) bottle of your favorite carrier oil, and shake the bottle well to disperse the oils thoroughly. Apply a few drops of your ready-to-use blend to sinus points around your nose and forehead, as well as on the back of your neck. You may repeat as needed.

Steam Inhalation to Support Respiratory System Formula

Steam inhalation with essential oils can be most effective for supporting the respiratory system and to aid in breathing. Whether you desire relief for asthma and allergy symptoms or for treating upper or lower respiratory tract infections, steam inhalation can be a great friend in your process of healing and recovery. Upper respiratory tract infections include sinusitis, tonsillitis, laryngitis and the common cold. Research now shows that poor oral hygiene and gum disease may be a contributing factor in pneumonia.

The essential oils in the respiratory support formula contain antibacterial, antihistamine, anti-allergic, antispasmodic and bronchodilating properties that make it useful for relieving respiratory conditions and associated symptoms of swelling and itching.

To a 5-ml, colored-glass, euro-dropper bottle add:

Blue Tansy: 20 drops

Hyssop: 20 drops

Frankincense: 20 drops

Lemon: 10 drops

Eucalyptus Radiata: 20 drops

Blue Yarrow: 10 drops

Close the cap tightly and shake the bottle vigorously to thoroughly blend the essential oils. Allow to synergize for 8 or more hours before using.

Use your Steam Inhalation Formula in a steam (refer to the "How to Use Essential Oils" section on page 20) or in a diffuser. Or you can dispense 1–3 drops of the respiratory blend onto a cotton ball or smell strip and inhale the aromatic vapors for 10–15 seconds. The formula is also effective as an aromatic mist. To make a ready-to-use blend, simply add 15–30 drops of your synergy blend to a 1-ounce (30-ml) bottle of your favorite carrier oil. Shake the bottle well to disperse the oils thoroughly. Apply a few drops of your ready-to-use blend to sinus points around your nose and forehead, as well as on the back of your neck. You may repeat as needed.

Oral Health Program

Complete Program for Prevention and Treatment of Tooth Decay and Gum Disease

For more than 10 years, I've practiced preventative dentistry and have used the treatments I recommend for preventing and reversing tooth decay, as well as whitening my teeth and keeping my gums healthy. Plus, I save money on dental care. When I went to my dentist for a cleaning recently, I had a full set of x-rays taken (the first I've had in 8 years). I wanted to check just in case I might have a cavity. My dentist, who supports my preventative dental care approach, gave my teeth a clean bill of health.

It is a common presumption that once you have a cavity the only way to "cure" it is to have a dentist drill out your cavity and replace it with a filling made of synthetic material. However, according to research that was published in the *British Medical Journal*, cavities and tooth decay can potentially be healed or even reversed with proper diet and nutrition.

When you remove the cause of cavities, your teeth naturally secrete new dentine to renew, repair and heal your teeth and gums. Your teeth thrive in an alkaline environment, so promoting alkalinity in your mouth through your diet and nutrition promotes the health of your teeth and gums.

I've used several different preventative dental care approaches and will share the program I've developed, which includes the use of a remineralizing toothpaste.

When a customer shared a type of remineralizing toothpaste recipe with me, I decided to give it a try myself. I adjusted the ingredients a little, so they were more to my own liking for a natural product.

After my first treatment, I noticed immediate results. I could actually feel and see a difference in the brightness of my smile and comfort level of my teeth and gums. Soon after beginning treatment, this natural remineralizing toothpaste had easily and effectively removed any signs of plaque buildup or stains from my teeth.

My teeth were noticeably whiter and brighter and felt stronger, healthier and happier. You know how your teeth feel after a good cleaning by the dental hygienist? That's how my teeth felt.

Oil Pulling

Oil pulling is a traditional folk remedy practiced in Ayurvedic medicine. Raw coconut oil contains 50 percent lauric acid, which the body converts into *monolaurin*, an antiviral, antibacterial and antiprotozoal agent that can destroy viruses like HIV, herpes, influenza and various other pathogens.

Oil pulling, or "oil swishing" as it is also called, is a method of swishing or holding the oil in the mouth for a period of time (20 minutes or longer). There are many claims for its improving oral and systemic health. It's thought to help various health issues like headache, migraine, asthma and acne, as well as to whiten the teeth. Oil swishing of coconut oil is thought to work by "pulling out" toxins.

Oil pulling is a part of my regular dental health routine. Coconut oil is a great cleanser and teeth whitener. I usually hold it in my mouth and swish it around for 30–60 minutes once a week between meals.

As part of my preventative dental program I also floss daily, brush with baking soda after meals and swish with hydrogen peroxide at least once daily. All have a therapeutically cleansing and whitening effect on the teeth and gums.

Natural Remineralizing Toothpaste Formula

This natural remineralizing toothpaste promotes removal of plaque buildup and stains.

Makes 8 ounces (237 ml):

¾ cup (175 ml) purified water, boiling

1 tbsp (15 ml) organic raw extra virgin coconut oil (kills viruses and bacteria)

¼ tsp Celtic salt (source of natural minerals)

½ tsp organic stevia leaf (green, unprocessed, dry herb and natural sweetener)

⅓ cup (75 g) bentonite green clay (draws out toxins and removes stains)

2 drops thyme oil (kills germs and bacteria, promotes healing of cavity)

2 drops oregano oil (kills germs and bacteria, promotes healing of cavity)

2 drops lemon oil (kills germs and bacteria, promotes healing of cavity)

2 drops cinnamon leaf oil (kills germs and bacteria, promotes healing of cavity)

2 drops clove bud oil (kills germs and bacteria, promotes healing of cavity)

15 drops peppermint oil (breath freshener)

In a pan, bring the water to a boil. In a ceramic bowl, add ¼ cup (60 ml) of the boiling water. Stir in the organic raw extra virgin coconut oil. Blend the Celtic salt and stevia into the liquid.

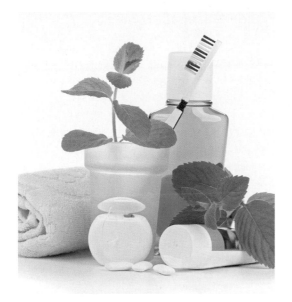

Recovery After Illness Formula

A powerful tonic, astringent and immune stimulant, this Recovery After Illness Formula contains essential oils with properties known for boosting and protecting the immune system. Its action to stimulate the formation of white blood cells aids the oxygenation of tissue and the removal of toxic waste. It may be effective for restoring the immune system after prolonged illness.

To a 5-ml, colored-glass, euro-dropper bottle add:
Geranium Roseum and Graveolens: 10 drops each
Myrrh: 20 drops
Frankincense: 20 drops
Lemon: 5 drops
Eucalyptus Globulus: 5 drops
Eucalyptus Radiata: 5 drops
Thyme: 5 drops
Lavender: 5 drops
Rosemary: 5 drops
Cypress: 5 drops
Ledum: 5 drops

Mix the bentonite clay into the hot liquid with a stainless steel spoon. Blend the mixture together until smooth and even like a paste. Add more heated purified water if needed to make a nice smooth and consistent paste. Blend the essential oils into the paste.

Transfer the remineralizing toothpaste into an 8-ounce (237-ml) glass container and seal tightly with a lid. Store in a cool, dark place.

To use, wet your toothbrush and dip the bristles onto the surface of the remineralizing toothpaste. Apply a sufficient amount of toothpaste to brush your teeth. Be sure to thoroughly brush each tooth. I recommend that you floss before brushing. Use daily until you finish the entire 8-ounce (237-ml) jar. Continue use as needed.

CAUTION: Oregano oil is a potent, "hot" antimicrobial and should be used with extreme caution. As it is a strong irritant to the skin and mucous membranes, use a less than 1 percent dilution for safe skin application. Avoid during pregnancy and with young children and pets.

Close the cap tightly and shake the bottle vigorously to thoroughly blend the essential oils. Allow to synergize for 8 or more hours before using.

Use in a diffuser or dispense 1–3 drops of the Recovery After Illness Formula onto a cotton ball or smell strip and inhale the aromatic vapors for 10–15 seconds. It is also effective as an aromatic mist. To make a ready-to-use Recovery After Illness blend, simply add 15–30 drops of your synergy blend to a 1-ounce (30-ml) bottle of your favorite carrier oil. Shake the bottle well to disperse the oils thoroughly. Apply a few drops of your ready-to-use blend to sinus points around your nose and forehead, as well as on the back of your neck. You may repeat as needed.

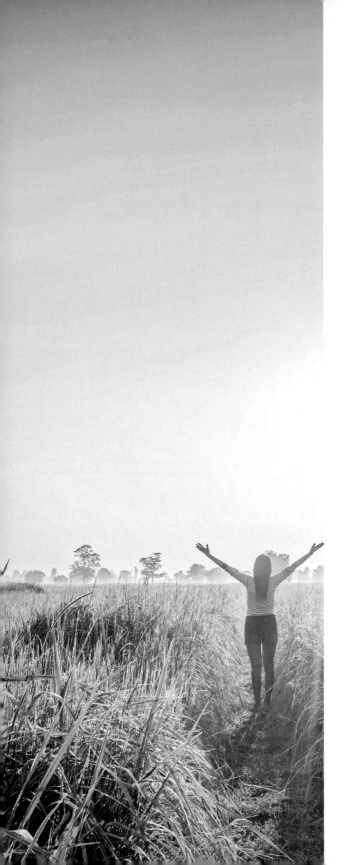

Rejuvenating and Healing Formula

A powerful, broad-spectrum tonic and immune stimulant, this Rejuvenating and Healing blend has tremendous capacity for healing. It contains nature's most potent antimicrobial oils for supporting and protecting the immune system, as well as killing viral, bacterial (especially airborne) and fungal infections.

To a 5-ml, colored-glass, euro-dropper bottle add:

Clove: 10 drops

Cinnamon Leaf: 10 drops

Eucalyptus Radiata: 20 drops

Lemon: 20 drops

Thyme: 5 drops

Oregano: 10 drops

Tea Tree: 5 drops

Lavender: 5 drops

Myrrh: 10 drops

Rosemary: 5 drops

Close the cap tightly and shake the bottle vigorously to thoroughly blend the essential oils. Allow to synergize for 8 or more hours before using.

Use in a diffuser, or dispense 1–3 drops of the Rejuvenating and Healing Formula onto a cotton ball or smell strip and inhale the aromatic vapors for 10–15 seconds. This formula is also effective as an aromatic mist. To make a ready-to-use Rejuvenating and Healing blend, simply add 15–30 drops of your synergy blend to a 1-ounce (30-ml) bottle of your favorite carrier oil. Shake the bottle well to disperse the oils thoroughly. Apply a few drops of your ready-to-use blend to sinus points around your nose and forehead, as well as on the back of your neck. You may repeat as needed.

Women's Health Formulas

These women's health formulas are the result of years of experience and working with women to help them find pure and natural solutions to their health concerns.

Female Toner

The female psyche is very open and sensitive to the environment and its influences. Being in the world can deplete energy reserves that need daily replenishing with sufficient rest and recovery time. Hormonal balance plays a crucial role in a woman's sense of well-being, level of emotional comfort and security. Nourishing the hormonal system with proper nutrition, exercise and time for rest and recovery helps to keep the hormonal system naturally balanced.

The essential oils in this Female Toner formula have been shown to have a regulating and balancing effect on the hormonal system and are helpful for relieving symptoms of imbalance like menstrual tension and cramping, as well as menopausal symptoms like hot flashes, headache, sleeplessness, tearfulness, depression, irritability and mood swings.

To a 5-ml, colored-glass, euro-dropper bottle add:

Geranium (Bourbon): 20 drops

Palmarosa: 20 drops

Lavender: 20 drops

Cypress: 20 drops

Clary Sage: 10 drops

Rose: 5 drops

Frankincense: 5 drops

Close the cap tightly and shake the bottle vigorously to thoroughly blend the essential oils. Allow to synergize for 8 or more hours before using.

Dispense 1–3 drops on a cotton ball or smell strip and inhale the aromatic vapors of your Female Toner for 10–15 seconds. You may repeat as needed. Female Toner may be especially effective used as a hot compress to relieve menstrual cramps.

To make a ready-to-use Female Toner blend simply add 15–30 drops of your synergy blend to a 1-ounce (30-ml) bottle of your favorite carrier oil. Shake the bottle well to disperse the oils thoroughly. Apply a few drops of your blend to sinus points around your nose and forehead, as well as on the back of your neck. Clients report that with regular use signs of hormonal imbalance diminish in severity and are less frequent or even stop completely.

Hormone Balance Formula

The endocrine glands secrete hormones (electrochemicals) that regulate all the body's organs and systems. Some of the body functions that hormones control include digestion, metabolism, respiration, perception, sleep, excretion, lactation, stress, growth and development, movement, reproduction and mood. Nourishing the hormonal system with proper nutrition, exercise and time for rest and recovery helps to keep the hormonal system naturally balanced.

The essential oils in this Hormone Balance Formula have been shown to have a regulating and balancing effect on the hormonal system and are helpful for relieving symptoms of imbalance like premenstrual tension and cramping, as well as menopausal symptoms like hot flashes, headache, sleeplessness, tearfulness, depression, irritability and mood swings.

(continued)

To a 5-ml, colored-glass, euro-dropper bottle add:

Geranium Graveolens: 20 drops

Palmarosa: 20 drops

Geranium Roseum: 20 drops

Clary Sage: 20 drops

Bergamot: 20 drops

Close the cap tightly and shake the bottle vigorously to thoroughly blend the essential oils. Allow to synergize for 8 or more hours before using.

Dispense 1–3 drops on a cotton ball or smell strip and inhale the aromatic vapors of your Hormone Balance Formula for 10–15 seconds. You may repeat as needed. This is also effective when diffused into the air or used as an aromatic mist.

To make a ready-to-use Hormone Balance Formula, simply add 15–30 drops of your synergy blend to a 1-ounce (30-ml) bottle of your favorite carrier oil. Shake the bottle well to disperse the oils thoroughly. Apply a few drops of your ready-to-use blend to sinus points around your nose and forehead, as well as on the back of your neck. Clients report that with regular use signs of hormonal imbalance diminish in severity, occur less frequently or even stop completely.

Hot Flash Relief Formula

Hot flashes are caused by fluctuations in hormones and are often associated with menopause. Symptoms include sudden intense heat, profuse sweating, visible reddening of the skin, feelings of faintness and rapid pulse. Symptoms can last for a couple of minutes or up to half an hour. Hot flashes may occur sporadically or be a common occurrence and disrupt the quality of one's life. Accompanying symptoms include night sweats (which interrupt sleep), insomnia, depression, poor mood and an inability to focus and pay attention.

The North American Menopause Society (NAMS) attributes certain foods and lifestyle habits to the aggravation of hot flashes, including hot and spicy foods, alcohol and caffeine. It's also thought that obesity issues may contribute to menopausal symptoms like hot flashes.

The essential oils in this formula have been shown to be effective as a comfort care measure to promote natural relief for symptoms of hot flashes.

To a 5-ml, colored-glass, euro-dropper bottle add:

Peppermint: 20 drops

Cypress: 20 drops

Lemon: 20 drops

Geranium Roseum and Graveolens: 5 drops each

Clary Sage: 10 drops

Palmarosa: 10 drops

Lemongrass: 10 drops

Cap the bottle tightly and shake vigorously to blend the essential oils. Allow to synergize for 8 hours or longer before using.

This formula makes a wonderfully cooling aromatic mist and is also effective diffused into the air. You may use as often as needed.

To make a ready-to-use Hot Flash Relief Formula, simply add 15–30 drops of your synergy blend to a 1-ounce (30-ml) bottle of your favorite carrier oil. Shake the bottle well to disperse the oils thoroughly. Apply a few drops of your ready-to-use blend to sinus points around your nose and forehead, as well as the back of your neck. Clients report that with regular use signs of hormonal imbalance like hot flashes diminish in severity, occur less frequently or even stop completely.

Breast Health

Breast self-awareness includes regular breast self-examination (BSE), a screening method used to detect early breast cancer. A BSE involves looking at and feeling each breast for painful or swollen tissue or any distortions in tissue quality.

Though much less commonly, men can develop breast cancer. So breast self-awareness is not gender-specific.

A regular breast massage is a great way to develop your breast self-awareness, as well as perform your BSE.

Why Performing a Regular Breast Massage Is So Beneficial

- Breast massage increases your personal awareness about changes in your breasts and is considered one of the most important methods for detection of breast cancer in its early stages.
- Breast massage sends an important message of self-love and acceptance, which is fundamental to good health.
- Breast massage allows you to learn to recognize and get comfortable with normal breast changes that may include natural lumpiness of your breast tissue.
- Breast massage increases the flow of lymph drainage to remove toxins within and around the breast, encouraging the area to remain free of toxic build-up. Lymph also carries immune cells for fighting against infection and rogue tissue growth, like cancer. Unlike the circulatory system, which has the heart to pump blood, the lymph system does not have a pump to move its fluids. The continuous action of muscular contraction squeezes lymph vessels to move lymph fluid throughout the lymphatic system. If there is prolonged restriction or tightness of tissues, lymph builds up and inflammation can occur.

- Much research supports the idea that when women wear bras they restrict the normal flow of lymph fluid within the breast tissue. Because the lymphatic system is responsible for the removal of toxins from your body, researchers have concluded that restricting the flow of lymph has the potential for contributing to the development of breast cancer, as well as other uncomfortable breast tissue conditions.
- To ensure healthy lymph flow and drainage and to promote healthy breast tissue, regular movement, exercise and stretching are absolutely essential. It is also important to practice breast health care with a regular BSE, which can include giving yourself a regular breast massage.

Breast Massage May Relieve These Symptoms:

- Breast tenderness
- Uneven or lumpy breast tissue
- Pre-menstrual tension and discomfort
- Swelling and pain from breast surgery
- Pectoralis muscle pain
- Mastitis

PLEASE NOTE: Your open readiness to discuss any unusual breast tissue changes you may find with your doctor is also very important.

Breast Health Massage Formula

The essential oils in this Breast Health Massage Formula have been shown to be effective for relieving symptoms of nausea that may be caused by dizziness, sea sickness, motion sickness, migraine headache, stomach flu or food poisoning. The formula also offers relief from nausea resulting from side effects of many medications, including chemotherapy, as well as morning sickness in early pregnancy.

The essential oils in the Breast Health Massage Formula promote gentle penetrating action that is regenerative and healing to breast tissue.

Gently apply a small amount of the Breast Health Massage Formula onto your breast and chest areas and lightly massage in, or use in a hot compress to help relieve congestion, promote circulation and relieve acute and chronic pain.

This massage oil also makes an excellent Swedish or deep tissue massage lubricant. You may use this oil during or after subtle bodywork, such as acupuncture, Reiki or Therapeutic Touch to enhance your treatment results.

To a 5-ml, colored-glass, euro-dropper bottle add:

Peppermint: 20 drops

Ginger: 20 drops

Lemon: 20 drops

Geranium Roseum: 30 drops

Clary Sage: 10 drops

Cap the bottle tightly and shake vigorously to blend the essential oils. Allow to synergize for 8 hours or longer before using.

To make a ready-to-use breast massage oil simply add 15–30 drops of your synergy blend to a 1-ounce (30-ml) bottle of your favorite carrier oil. Shake the bottle well to disperse the oils thoroughly. Dispense 1–3 drops. Inhale the scent of the oil first and then apply to the breast and massage thoroughly into the tissues.

Fibroids Formula

"True health is only possible when we understand the unity of our minds, emotions, spirits and physical bodies and stop striving for perfection." —Christiane Northrup, MD

Uterine fibroids are considered benign tumors of the uterus. The medical term for a fibroid tumor is *myoma* or *fibromyoma*. Up to 80 percent of women develop fibroids by age fifty. In 2013 it was reported that 171 million women had fibroids. Fibroids are most often asymptomatic, depending upon their size and location. Symptoms may include heavy periods and frequent urination, as well as occasionally a hindrance for getting pregnant.

Though the cause of fibroids isn't clear, the tendency for getting a fibroid seems genetically linked and can run in one's family. Obesity and overeating, especially red meat, also seem to be causative factors.

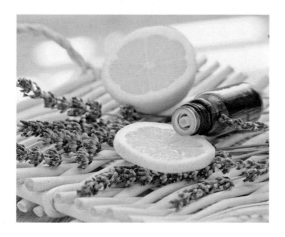

Dr. Christiane Northrup, an OB/GYN physician for 25 years and the author of *Women's Bodies, Women's Wisdom*, says that many women develop uterine fibroids during the middle and later reproductive years. After menopause, fibroids usually decrease in size and even disappear. The research seems to bear this out. However, in the U.S., uterine fibroids are a common reason for surgical removal of the uterus.

The essential oils in this comfort care formula have been shown to be effective for relieving fibroid symptoms.

To a 5-ml, colored-glass, euro-dropper bottle add:

Lavender: 20 drops

Lemon: 10 drops

Juniper Berry: 10 drops

Palmarosa: 40 drops

Helichrysum: 20 drops

Cap the bottle tightly and shake vigorously to blend the essential oils. Allow to synergize for 8 hours or longer before using. To get the best results, use this formula in a sitz bath.

Sitz Bath

A sitz bath will help you focus your essential oil treatment to the area of discomfort for better results.

1–3 cups (500–1,500 g) Epsom or sea salts

15–18 drops Fibroids Formula

Pour the salts into a bowl and add the Fibroids Formula essential oils blend. Blend together thoroughly. Cover and set aside.

Fill the sitz bath with pure warm water (98°F [37°C]), add the scented salts and blend in thoroughly. Soak in the bath for 15 minutes or until the waters cool. Repeat as needed to relieve symptoms of discomfort and to support natural healing. This formula is also effective as a warm compress over the lower belly or any area of discomfort.

You can also use a sitz bath for other treatments like for Bartholin gland cysts. A sitz bath is more effective for getting results than a full bath.

To ensure the essential oils are absorbed into the salts, it's now recommended that the oils are first added to 1 teaspoon unscented liquid soap, like Castile for example, or other unscented natural liquid soap, before adding to sea salts.

CHAPTER 10

Relaxation and Emotional Support Formulas

Enthusiasm

When one is filled with an intense enjoyment of life and the feeling of being alive, there is nothing one cannot do. You look forward to each day with renewed optimism and faith in the unseen adventures life will bring you. Many children are quite naturally filled with an enthusiastic spirit and throw themselves into every activity with wild abandon. The word "enthusiastic" was first coined by the Greeks and meant "possessed by god's essence." If you've lost your zest for life, essential oils can help renew and lift your spirits.

Lift the Spirits Formula

This Lift the Spirits Formula contains essential oils with stimulating, regulating and energizing properties that make it effective for lifting your spirits and renewing your enthusiasm for life.

To a 5-ml, colored-glass, euro-dropper bottle add:

Grapefruit: 40 drops

Peppermint: 20 drops

Lemon: 20 drops

Geranium Roseum and Graveolens: 10 drops each

Close the cap tightly and shake the bottle vigorously to thoroughly blend the essential oils. Allow to synergize for 8 or more hours before using.

Dispense 1–3 drops on a cotton ball or smell strip and inhale the aromatic vapors of your Lift the Spirits Formula for 10–15 seconds. You may repeat as needed. This formula is also effective when diffused into the air, as an aromatic mist or in the bath.

To make a ready-to-use Lift the Spirits Formula, simply add 15–30 drops of your synergy blend to a 1-ounce (30-ml) bottle of your favorite carrier oil. Shake the bottle well to disperse the oils thoroughly. Apply a few drops of your ready-to-use blend to sinus points around your nose and forehead, as well as on the back of your neck.

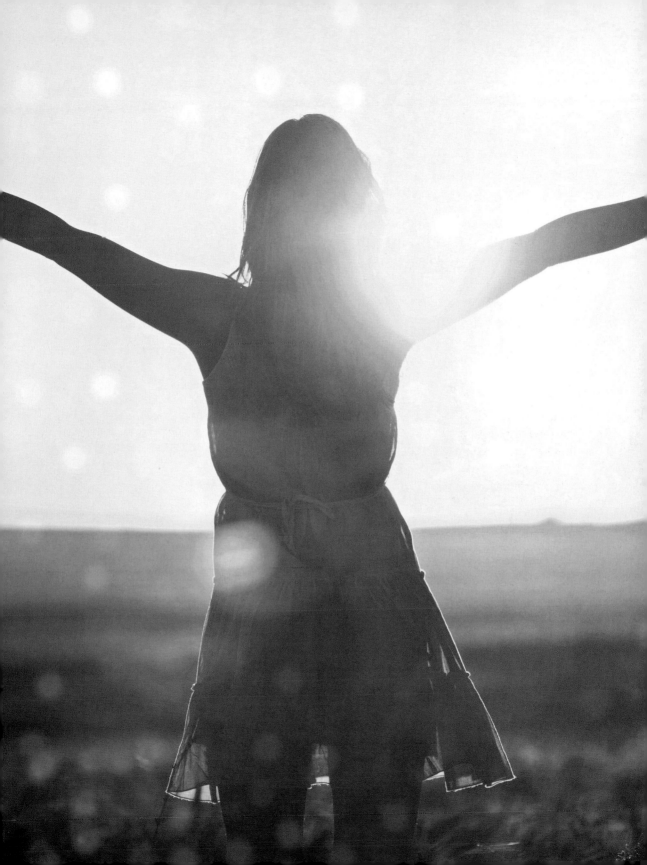

Mood

A mood is a very general emotional state that can dramatically affect how you experience life. When you're in a good mood, things seem to go your way. Whereas, when you're in a bad mood, it can feel like you have two left feet and can't seem to get in sync with your life. Sometimes you just wake up in a bad mood or something happens that triggers a bad mood. Essential oils are great for creating an ambiance that will immediately shift a bad mood—or enhance an already good one—so that you feel even better almost instantly.

Lift the Mood Formula

This Lift the Mood Formula contains essential oils with regulating properties that may be effective for shifting mental states and lifting the mood.

To a 5-ml, colored-glass, euro-dropper bottle add:

Bergamot: 40 drops

Ylang Ylang III: 20 drops

Geranium Roseum and Graveolens: 10 drops each

Clary Sage: 20 drops

Close the cap tightly and shake the bottle vigorously to thoroughly blend the essential oils. Allow to synergize for 8 or more hours before using.

Dispense 1–3 drops on a cotton ball or smell strip and inhale the aromatic vapors of your Lift the Mood blend for 10–15 seconds. You may repeat as needed. This formula is also effective when diffused into the air, as an aromatic mist or in the bath.

To make a ready-to-use Lift the Mood Formula, simply add 15–30 drops of your synergy blend to a 1-ounce (30-ml) bottle of your favorite carrier oil. Shake the bottle well to disperse the oils thoroughly. Apply a few drops of your ready-to-use blend to sinus points around your nose and forehead, as well as on the back of your neck.

Meditation

Some form of meditation or mindfulness practice has been around since antiquity. Meditation may include many different practices and techniques for the purpose of calming and regulating the mind, as well as recognizing a heightened state of awareness. Becoming identified with pure consciousness while doing some form of meditation helps to free the meditator from the grip of the egoism of the mind, which is changeable and thus a source of suffering. Many health problems are now being treated with meditation, including high blood pressure, depression and anxiety. Meditation is also used to engender loving kindness and compassion for one's fellow man.

Meditation Formula

The essential oils in the Meditation Formula support a meditation practice by calming and harmonizing your mind and emotions and slowing down your heart rate, breathing and cellular respiration.

To a 5-ml, colored-glass, euro-dropper bottle add:

Frankincense: 20 drops

Atlas Cedarwood: 20 drops

Myrrh: 20 drops

Spikenard: 20 drops

Ylang Ylang III: 10 drops

Bergamot: 10 drops

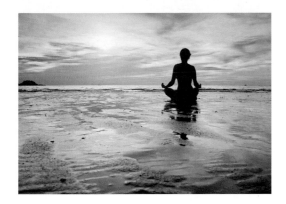

Close the cap tightly and shake the bottle vigorously to thoroughly blend the essential oils. Allow to synergize for 8 or more hours before using.

Dispense 1–3 drops on a cotton ball or smell strip and inhale the aromatic vapors of your meditation blend for 10–15 seconds. You may repeat as needed. This formula is also effective when diffused into the air or as an aromatic mist.

To make a ready-to-use Meditation Formula blend, simply add 15–30 drops of your synergy blend to a 1-ounce (30-ml) bottle of your favorite carrier oil. Shake the bottle well to disperse the oils thoroughly. Apply a few drops to sinus points around your nose and forehead, as well as on the back of your neck.

Stress Relief

The strain, effort and pressure induced by the demands of stress can be good in that stress provides an incredible stimulus to grow and reach new potentials for oneself, whether physically or psychologically. However, ongoing and long-term stress can also have a damaging effect with attributes that may be less than desirable, leading to anxiety, stroke, ulcers, heart attack, depression and nervous disorders. Essential oils can help relieve stress, as well as help you handle it better.

Stress Relief Formula

This Stress Relief Formula contains essential oils with powerful sedative action, helping to calm the emotions and an overactive and turbulent mind.

To a 5-ml, colored-glass, euro-dropper bottle add:
Vetiver: 20 drops
Spikenard: 20 drops
Chamomile: 20 drops
Geranium Roseum and Graveolens: 10 drops each
Clary Sage: 20 drops

Close the cap tightly and shake the bottle vigorously to thoroughly blend the essential oils. Allow to synergize for 8 or more hours before using.

Dispense 1–3 drops on a cotton ball or smell strip and inhale the aromatic vapors of your Stress Relief Formula for 10–15 seconds. You may repeat as needed. This formula is also effective when diffused into the air, as an aromatic mist or in the bath.

To make a ready-to-use Stress Relief Formula blend, simply add 15–30 drops of your synergy blend to a 1-ounce (30-ml) bottle of your favorite carrier oil. Shake the bottle well to disperse the oils thoroughly. Apply a few drops to sinus points around your nose and forehead, as well as on the back of your neck.

Anxiety Relief

Anxiety is a kind of fearful expectation about the future that comes from a turbulent inner mind that worries and imagines what might go wrong. It is not based on a real event that is happening but is rather the imagination running wild. It's an unpleasant state of mind that can lead to feelings of dread about what might happen in the future. Physical symptoms often accompany anxiety, such as heart palpitations, hair loss, insomnia, aches and pains, irritable bowel, OCD, loss of appetite, restlessness and an inability to focus. Everyone experiences anxiety periodically. Essential oils can help relieve simple anxiety and its related symptoms.

Anxiety Relief Formula

Helpful for letting go of stressful emotions and soothing an overactive, troubled or nervous state of mind, the essential oils in the Anxiety Relief Formula are known for their sedative action and ability to promote inner balance, peace and calm.

To a 5-ml, colored-glass, euro-dropper bottle add:

Red Mandarin: 20 drops

Bergamot: 20 drops

Ylang Ylang III: 20 drops

German Chamomile: 10 drops

Roman Chamomile: 10 drops

Spikenard: 10 drops

Vetiver: 10 drops

Close the cap tightly and shake the bottle vigorously to thoroughly blend the essential oils. Allow to synergize for 8 or more hours before using.

Dispense 1–3 drops on a cotton ball or smell strip and inhale the aromatic vapors of your Anxiety Relief Formula for 10–15 seconds. You may repeat as needed. This formula is also effective when diffused into the air or as an aromatic mist.

To make a ready-to-use Anxiety Relief Formula blend, simply add 15–30 drops of your synergy blend to a 1-ounce (30-ml) bottle of your favorite carrier oil. Shake the bottle well to disperse the oils thoroughly. Apply a few drops to sinus points around your nose and forehead, as well as on the back of your neck

Depression Relief

When a person is depressed, they experience a lowered state of mood, which affects their thoughts, feelings, behaviors and overall sense of well-being. Depression can express itself in many different ways, including feelings of sadness, anxiety, hopelessness, guilt, shame, low self-worth, loss of appetite or overeating, insomnia or sleeplessness, poor ability to focus, body aches and pain, poor digestion and low energy.

Research is showing that depression can be inherited through one's cultural conditioning and early childhood experiences. Certain medications or even foods like sugar can lead to a letdown withdrawal response that lowers the mood. Life events like the death of a loved one, the loss of a job, physical illness, a major life transition (like puberty or menopause) or feelings like anger can all contribute to depression. Depression can lead to withdrawal from daily activities and isolation from others.

Depression is most often a temporary and natural state that both men and women can experience in life at one time or another. When you accept and allow yourself to feel your feelings, you can pass on through them. Feelings are not one's identity, but rather a transitory experience everyone has. Essential oils can be used as a comfort care measure to help lift the mood and promote a happier state of mind.

Depression Relief Formula 1

This formula will help lift your mood and shift you to a more positive mental state.

To a 5-ml, colored-glass, euro-dropper bottle add:

Lemon: 10 drops

Tangerine: 20 drops

Sweet Orange: 10 drops

Bergamot: 20 drops

Ylang Ylang: 20 drops

Geranium: 20 drops

Cap the bottle tightly and shake vigorously to blend the essential oils. Allow to synergize for 8 hours or longer before using.

Dispense 1–3 drops on a cotton ball or smell strip and inhale the aromatic vapors of your Depression Relief blend for 10–15 seconds. You may repeat as needed. This formula is also effective diffused into the air.

To make a ready-to-use Depression Relief Formula simply add 15–30 drops of your synergy blend to a 1-ounce (30-ml) bottle of your favorite carrier oil. Shake the bottle well to disperse the oils thoroughly. Dispense 1–3 drops, inhale the scent first and then apply behind both ears, as well as on the back of your neck.

Depression Relief Formula 2

A comforting and supportive tonic for your body, mind, spirit and emotions, the essential oils in the Depression Relief Formula contain properties that are known to calm the nerves, elevate the mood and relieve depressive states of mind.

To a 5-ml, colored-glass, euro-dropper bottle add:

Ylang Ylang III: 40 drops

Bergamot: 40 drops

Geranium Roseum and Graveolens: 5 drops each

Sweet Orange: 5 drops

Atlas Cedarwood: 5 drops

Close the cap tightly and shake the bottle vigorously to thoroughly blend the essential oils. Allow to synergize for 8 or more hours before using.

Dispense 1–3 drops on a cotton ball or smell strip and inhale the aromatic vapors of your Depression Relief Formula 2 blend for 10–15 seconds. You may repeat as needed. This formula is also effective when diffused into the air or as an aromatic mist.

To make a ready-to-use Depression Relief Formula 2 blend, simply add 15–30 drops of your synergy blend to a 1-ounce (30-ml) bottle of your favorite carrier oil. Shake the bottle well to disperse the oils thoroughly. Apply a few drops to sinus points around your nose and forehead, as well as on the back of your neck.

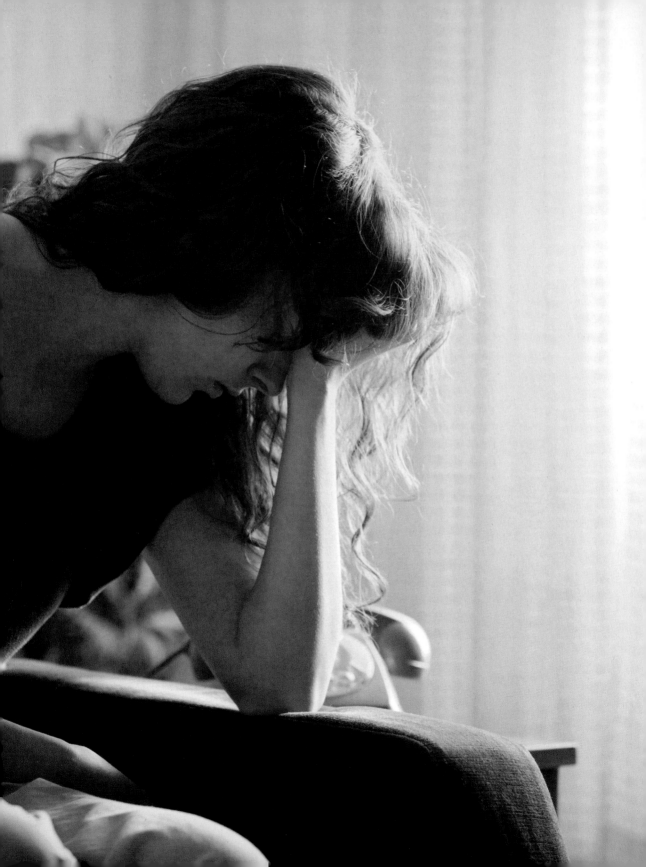

Grief and Loss

Bereavement for the loss of a loved one is a very complicated process that each of us experiences in life. In a world that is continually changing, there is always some form of loss occurring in each of our lives, especially the death or loss of someone or something we have loved whole-heartedly, and it can feel extremely painful. Bonds with loved ones, formed over many years, take time to release or move on to a new phase with. The feeling of loss can be so deep that it can be felt at all levels of our being—including our heart, mind, body and soul—in the routines of our daily life.

Grief and the loss it entails can be so pervasive that it can take time to process our loss and feel whole again. Essential oils can definitely play the role of a comforting friend. They can help with the process of grieving and letting go of a loved one and moving forward to the next stage in our life.

Grief and Loss Formula

This Grief and Loss Formula promotes the release of painful memories, regret, guilt, disappointment, anxiety, stress, emotional wounds and psychic tension. It may also be useful for overcoming addictions.

To a 5-ml, colored-glass, euro-dropper bottle add:

Red Mandarin: 20 drops

Ylang Ylang III: 20 drops

Frankincense: 20 drops

Geranium Roseum and Graveolens: 10 drops each

Bergamot: 10 drops

Helichrysum: 5 drops

Rose: 5 drops

Close the cap tightly and shake the bottle vigorously to thoroughly blend the essential oils. Allow to synergize for 8 or more hours before using.

Dispense 1–3 drops on a cotton ball or smell strip and inhale the aromatic vapors of your Grief and Loss Formula blend for 10–15 seconds. You may repeat as needed. This formula is also effective when diffused into the air, used in a bath or sprayed as an aromatic mist.

To make a ready-to-use Grief and Loss Formula blend, simply add 15–30 drops of your synergy blend to a 1-ounce (30-ml) bottle of your favorite carrier oil. Shake the bottle well to disperse the oils thoroughly. Apply a few drops to sinus points around your nose and forehead, as well as on the back of your neck.

CHAPTER 11

Spa and Beauty
Treatments

Complete Skincare Beauty Treatment Program

I have to admit that I never once saw anyone in my family perform any skincare routine. Never once do I recall seeing any hygienic routines for skincare even from my mom, who was a licensed cosmetologist and really into the idea of beauty. She was always buying the latest skin lotions, creams and make-up, but cleansing did not seem to be a part of her beauty care system.

It wasn't until I reached the age of thirty that it suddenly dawned on me that a regular facial cleansing ritual might be a good idea. At this same time, I started hydrating by drinking lots of pure fresh water. This was well before the bottled drinking craze that came along several years later.

As with all of my health routines and habits, my skincare treatment program has evolved for me intuitively and naturally over time. Periodically, I'll change things up a bit, but essentially this is the complete skincare beauty treatment program that I follow. By the way, I never use any body lotions on my skin. I used to, but not anymore. My diet has ample oils like raw extra virgin coconut and olive oils that nourish my skin from the inside so that it stays moist and supple.

For beautiful, healthy and radiant skin, try a skincare routine like this one, keeping in mind to use the skincare formulas that are right for your skin type.

- Skincare Formulas (once daily—page 105)
- Body and Facial Skin Toners (once daily, or as needed—page 108)
- French Clay Facial Mask (once monthly—page 110)
- Repair Butters for Body and Face (as needed—page 112)
- Hair and Scalp Treatments (once monthly—page 113)
- Lip Balms (once daily or as needed—page 116)
- Exfoliating Sugar Scrubs (before bath or shower—page 119)
- Salt Glow Treatments (once daily—page 120)

Skincare Formulas

Your skin, called the integumentary system, is your largest organ. It protects and guards the underlying muscles, bones, ligaments and internal organs.

The skin interacts with the external environment and is your first line of defense against external conditions. For instance, the skin plays a vital role in protecting the body against foreign invaders and guards against excessive water loss. It also functions as insulation to protect against heat loss, provides ventilation to keep you cool through perspiration and gives you experiences of both pleasurable and painful sensation.

Personally, I've made all of my own skincare products for more than 20 years and have not had any skin issues since that time. I used to be troubled with regular breakouts, which completely stopped after beginning to make my own skincare products. Sufficient hydration also plays a key role in healthy skin.

Skincare Formulas for Different Skin Types

For facial cleansing, I like to use raw, unscented, goat milk soap made fresh from the farm. If you are still washing your skin with soap made with a water base, then you're missing out on a truly great facial cleanser. It's certainly the best facial soap I've ever used to date. It is gentle, soothing and nourishing for your facial skin, and one bar lasts an incredibly long time. Raw goat's milk soap is beneficial for dry, sensitive, oily or problematic skin conditions like eczema and psoriasis or for keeping your skin healthy. I wash with either a hypoallergenic facial mitt made from flax (my preference) or a natural facial loofa to gently exfoliate my skin daily.

Normal to Dry Skincare Formula

Harmonizing for dry to normal skin types, the oils in this formula are known for their ability to tone, moisturize, balance and heal dry skin cells. Excellent for smoothing lines and wrinkles, use alone or add a drop to your favorite moisturizer or night cream.

To a 5-ml, colored-glass, euro-dropper bottle add:
Lavender: 10 drops
Geranium Roseum and Graveolens: 10 drops each
Palmarosa: 30 drops
Ylang Ylang: 40 drops

Close the cap tightly and shake the bottle vigorously to thoroughly blend the essential oils. Allow to synergize for 8 or more hours before using.

To make a ready-to-use Skincare Formula blend simply add 12–15 drops of your synergy blend to a 1-ounce (30-ml) bottle of your favorite carrier oil. Shake the bottle well to disperse the oils thoroughly. Apply 1–3 drops of your ready-to-use blend to your fingertips and gently apply to your face. Use upward sweeping motions to completely cover your skin. Very little is needed, and the oil should quickly absorb into your skin. If your skin feels oily or greasy after application, then you've used too much of the oil. Use once daily at the end of your regular facial cleansing routine.

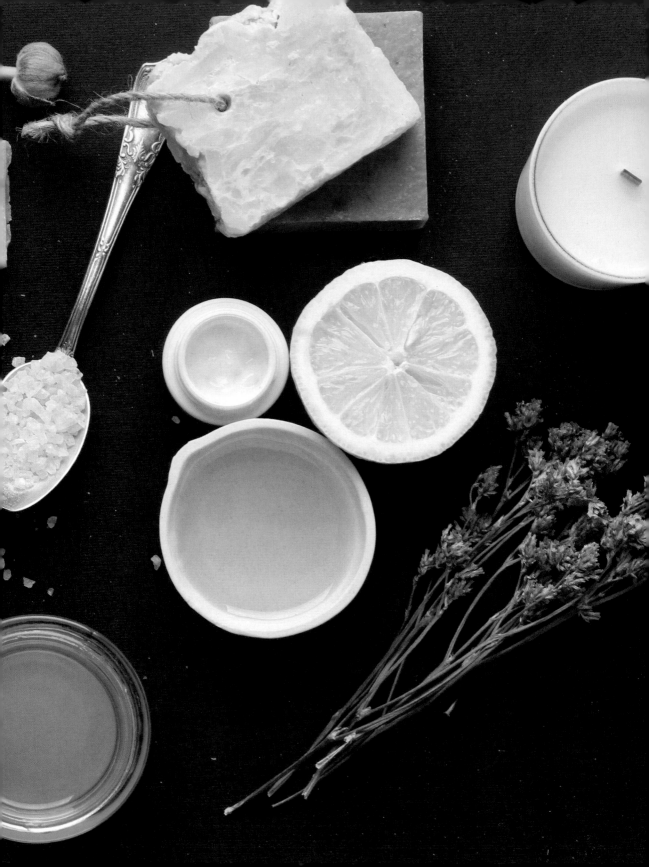

Oily Skincare Formula

This formula is harmonizing and balancing for oily skin cells. Use alone, or add a drop to your favorite skin care product.

To a 5-ml, colored-glass, euro-dropper bottle add:

Cypress: 40 drops

Myrrh: 10 drops

Carrot Seed: 10 drops

Geranium: 40 drops

Rosemary Verbenone: 1–2 drops

Close the cap tightly and shake the bottle vigorously to thoroughly blend the essential oils. Allow to synergize for 8 or more hours before using.

To make a ready-to-use skincare blend, simply add 12–15 drops of your synergy blend to a 1-ounce (30-ml) bottle of your favorite carrier oil. Shake the bottle well to disperse the oils thoroughly. Apply 1–3 drops of your ready-to-use blend to your fingertips and gently apply to your face. Use upward sweeping motions to completely cover your skin. Very little is needed, and the oil should quickly absorb into your skin. If your skin feels oily or greasy after application, then you've used too much of the oil. Use once daily at the end of your regular facial cleansing routine.

Sensitive Skincare Formula

Harmonizing for sensitive skin types, the oils in this formula are known for their ability to tone, moisturize, balance and heal sensitive skin cells. Use alone, or add a drop to your favorite moisturizer or night cream.

To a 5-ml, colored-glass, euro-dropper bottle add:

German Chamomile: 40 drops

Palmarosa: 30 drops

Rose: 10 drops

Helichrysum: 10 drops

Carrot Seed: 10 drops

Galbanum: 1–2 drops

Close the cap tightly and shake the bottle vigorously to thoroughly blend the essential oils. Allow to synergize for 8 or more hours before using.

To make a ready-to-use skincare blend, simply add 12–15 drops of your synergy blend to a 1-ounce (30-ml) bottle of your favorite carrier oil. Shake the bottle well to disperse the oils thoroughly. Apply 1–3 drops of your ready-to-use blend to your fingertips and gently apply to your face. Use upward sweeping motions to completely cover your skin. Very little is needed, and the oil should quickly absorb into your skin. If your skin feels oily or greasy after application, then you've used too much of the oil. Use once daily at the end of your regular facial cleansing routine.

Mature Skincare Formula

This blend is harmonizing and balancing for mature skin cells and excellent for smoothing and softening facial lines and wrinkles. Use alone or add a drop to your favorite moisturizer or night cream.

To a 5-ml, colored-glass, euro-dropper bottle add:

Frankincense: 20 drops

Rose: 20 drops

Ylang Ylang: 20 drops

Geranium Roseum and Graveolens: 10 drops each

Helichrysum: 10 drops

Carrot Seed: 10 drops

Close the cap tightly and shake the bottle vigorously to thoroughly blend the essential oils. Allow to synergize for 8 or more hours before using.

To make a ready-to-use skincare blend, simply add 12–15 drops of your synergy blend to a 1-ounce (30-ml) bottle of your favorite carrier oil. Shake the bottle well to disperse the oils thoroughly. Apply 1–3 drops of your ready-to-use blend to your fingertips and gently apply to your face. Use upward sweeping motions to completely cover your skin. Very little is needed, and the oil should quickly absorb into your skin. If your skin feels oily or greasy after application, then you've used too much of the oil. Use once daily at the end of your regular facial cleansing routine.

Body and Facial Skin Toners

A skin toner may be used for your body or face and is designed to cleanse and freshen your skin, as well as shrink the appearance of pores. You can use your body and facial toners by applying on cotton or to a damp woolen cloth, or you can spray directly on your face as a freshener.

Toner may be applied after your usual skin washing routine, and should be immediately followed by applying moisturizer once the toner has dried.

The mildest and most gentle form of skin toner that's suitable for all skin types, including dry and sensitive skin, uses pure fresh water and a small percentage of an astringent like alcohol or witch hazel (0–10 percent). Some kind of humectant like glycerin may also be used to hold in skin moisture, as well as to act as a preservative.

For slightly more skin-toning action that's suitable for all skin types, including oily and combination skin, use a bit more astringent (up to 20 percent) in water with a humectant, if desired.

Finally, the strongest toners are excellent for oily skin and controlling excess sebum production. These skin toners contain higher percentages of astringent (up to 60 percent) and the strongest antiseptic properties and action, which helps to prevent and control acne outbreaks.

Adding an essential oil or blend to your toner—that has skin nourishing and healing properties suitable for your skin type—enhances the effectiveness of your toner. Check out the section on skincare formulas (page 105) for different skin types and for more formulas to use in your toner.

Facial and Body Toner Formula (Normal to Dry Skin)

This may be used as a facial toner or as an allover body freshener.

I recommend the following essential oils by skin type and suitability for the particular skin condition as noted:

- German chamomile (sensitive skin)
- Geranium roseum and graveolens (regulating for all skin types)
- Palmarosa (problem skin)
- Lavender (burns and sunburned skin)
- Ylang ylang (moisturizing and balancing for all skin types)
- Cypress (oily skin)
- Myrrh and patchouli (dry, cracked and chapped skin)
- Frankincense (mature skin)
- Rose (mature skin; reduces appearance of lines and wrinkles)

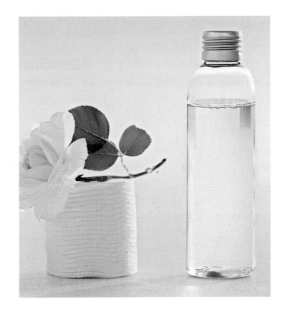

To a 5-ml, colored-glass, euro-dropper bottle add:

Lavender: 20 drops

Ylang Ylang III: 30 drops

Geranium Roseum and Graveolens: 25 drops each

1 (2-oz [60-ml]) colored-glass misting bottle

1 tsp glycerin (optional)

Astringent (alcohol or witch hazel, 0–20 percent)

8–12 drops essential oil or blend by skin type

Purified or fresh spring water

Close the cap of the euro-dropper bottle tightly and shake the bottle vigorously to thoroughly blend the essential oils. Allow to synergize for 8 or more hours before using.

To a 2-ounce (60-ml), colored-glass misting bottle, add your teaspoon of glycerin (if you're using it). Next, add the astringent to the bottle, cap with the atomizer top and shake the bottle vigorously to mix the glycerin and astringent. Add the essential oil or blend to the mixture, cap the bottle again and shake vigorously to blend the oils in the mixture. Add water to fill the bottle, making sure to leave room to insert the atomizer spray top.

As there is no true emulsifying agent in this recipe, the oils will not stay completely mixed with the glycerin, astringent and water, so you will need to shake the bottle well each time before using.

Use your facial and body toner any time. You may find it especially beneficial after your shower, bath or facial cleansing ritual. Lightly spray onto the desired skin areas to freshen, heal and tone. You may also spray toner onto a cotton or woolen pad and apply to your face and skin with gentle, upward, sweeping movements. Allow to dry thoroughly before applying a facial moisturizer or body lotion, if desired.

French Clay Facial Mask

Use this clay facial mask formula made with French clay and essential oils to promote cleansing and detoxification of your facial skin, as well as to improve your skin's elasticity and impart a radiant, healthy glow. Create a supportive and relaxing environment for enjoying and making the most of your time by turning off phones and electronic devices. Make the room comfortably warm for relaxing during and for a brief time after your facial mask. Light a candle and play gentle and soothing music in the background, or just relax and be still during and after your treatment.

Rose: 30 drops (You can use a 10 percent dilution in carrier oil. If you use rose oil that has been diluted in a carrier oil, be sure to wait and add it directly to the French clay mixture, because a diluted essential oil will not synergize with other essential oils and can prevent other oils from synergizing with each other.)

Geranium Roseum and Graveolens: 20 drops each

Ylang Ylang: 20 drops

Carrot Seed: 10 drops

1 tbsp (15 g) French pink or green clay

1½–2 tbsp (22–30 ml) purified or spring water or cream

⅛ tsp light coconut oil or other suitable vegetable oil of your choice (Refer to the "Face Carrier Oils" section on page 25 for more about carrier oils.)

Make a synergy blend of your essential oils in a 5-milliliter euro-dropper bottle and allow to synergize for a minimum of 24 hours. Refer to the "Aromatherapy Blending Guide" on page 48 for more about making synergy blends.

Before preparing your facial mask, wash your face with your favorite cleanser and towel dry.

In a small bowl, mix together your choice of natural French clay with the purified or spring water (or cream) and the light coconut oil to make a loose paste, but make sure it's not wet.

Add one drop of the essential oil synergy blend to the paste and blend thoroughly together.

Immediately begin applying the French Clay Facial Mask to your face using gentle upward sweeping strokes. Start with your décolletage and apply the mask evenly over your chin, both cheeks, nose and forehead. Be sure to completely cover your entire face with the mask.

After applying the mask and completely covering your face with it, take time to relax. Enjoy a refreshing glass of water with a slice of lemon as you allow the mask to dry for 10–20 minutes.

Rinse off your facial mask thoroughly with warm water, making sure the mask is completely removed. Your skin will feel soft, silky smooth, toned and refreshed. After your facial mask, you can perform your usual cleansing and moisturizing routine if you like and continue to hydrate with fresh-squeezed lemon water.

CAUTION: Clay may stain fabric, so take care.

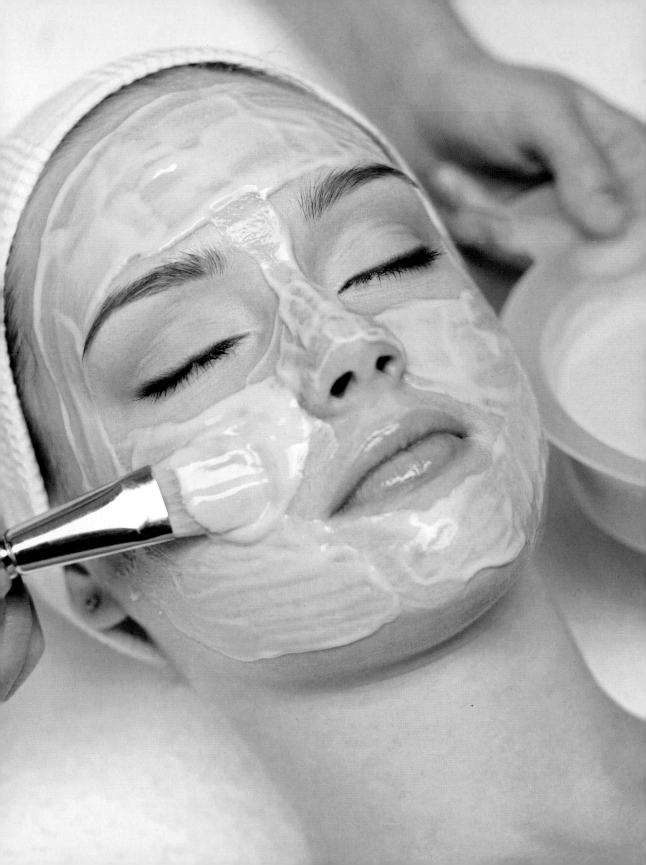

Repair Butters for Body and Face

Repair butter is excellent for moisturizing and deep healing of skin cell tissue. Use on body parts that are weathered, dry, cracked or chapped, like the soles of feet and heels or to areas that have signs of premature aging such as face lines and wrinkles. When applied topically on skin, the waxy substance of this regenerative repair butter acts as an intensive, long-wear protective barrier to the elements. It also helps to moisturize and heal the skin.

Repair Butter Essential Oils Formula

This non-greasy and petroleum-free repair butter is formulated to moisturize and heal aging, dry or cracked skin. It's easy to make, with the addition of shea or cocoa butter, which boosts its moisturizing capacity. It can be stored for periods of a year or longer when vitamin E oil is used as a natural preservative and the butter is sealed properly and stored in the refrigerator.

Makes a 1-ounce (30-ml) container of repair butter:

1 tbsp (21 g) beeswax (Less beeswax makes your butter softer and more gives it a firmer consistency.)

1 tbsp (15 g) shea or cocoa butter

¼ cup (60 ml) light coconut oil

30–36 drops any essential oil synergy blend

4 drops vitamin E oil

Put the beeswax and shea butter into the light coconut oil and heat in a double boiler. For a homemade double boiler, use a glass measuring cup (such as Pyrex) inside a pan of water. Heat the mixture over medium-low heat until the beeswax and shea butter melt.

Remove from the heat source and allow the liquid to cool slightly before adding your essential oil synergy blend. Gently blend in the oils with a sterile instrument. Add the vitamin E oil. Immediately pour the mixture into a 1-ounce (30-ml) container and refrigerate, allowing to cool.

Apply the repair butter liberally with your fingertips to problem areas of your skin to moisturize and heal skin tissues. Use as frequently as you like; it won't build up!

Premature Aging Skincare Formula

Regulating and harmonizing action for skin cells, this formula is known for its toning and moisturizing ability. Use alone, or add a drop to your favorite moisturizer.

To a 5-ml, colored-glass, euro-dropper bottle add:

Geranium Roseum and Graveolens: 20 drops each

Rose: 30 drops

Ylang Ylang: 30 drops

Close the cap tightly and shake the bottle vigorously to thoroughly blend the essential oils. Allow to synergize for 8 or more hours before using.

To make a ready-to-use skincare blend, simply add 12–15 drops of your synergy blend to a 1-ounce (30-ml) bottle of your favorite carrier oil. Shake the bottle well to disperse the oils thoroughly. Apply 1–3 drops of your blend to your fingertips and gently apply to your face. Use upward sweeping motions to completely cover your skin. Very little is needed, and the oil should quickly absorb into your skin. If your skin feels oily or greasy after application, then you've used too much of the oil. Use once daily at the end of your regular facial cleansing routine.

Severely Dry and Cracked Skin Formula

This blend is harmonizing and balancing for severely cracked and dry skin cell tissues. Use alone or add a drop to your favorite moisturizer or night cream.

To a 5-ml, colored-glass, euro-dropper bottle add:

Myrrh: 50 drops

Spikenard: 30 drops

Helichrysum: 20 drops

Close the cap tightly and shake the bottle vigorously to thoroughly blend the essential oils. Allow to synergize for 8 or more hours before using.

To make a ready-to-use skincare blend, simply add 12–15 drops of your synergy blend to a 1-ounce (30-ml) bottle of your favorite carrier oil. Shake the bottle well to disperse the oils thoroughly. Apply 1–3 drops of your blend to your fingertips and gently apply to your face. Use upward sweeping motions to completely cover your skin. Very little is needed, and the oil should quickly absorb into your skin. If your skin feels oily or greasy after application, then you've used too much of the oil. Use once daily at the end of your regular facial cleansing routine.

Hair and Scalp Treatments

The condition of your hair is largely dependent upon a good supply of blood carrying adequate amounts of nutrition such as amino acids, vitamins and minerals to your hair follicle. Your hair is made of keratin, a stretchable protein material manufactured by your hair follicle. Hair follicles in your scalp grow at a rate of about half an inch (1.3 cm) per month, though this rate of growth can vary.

An aromatherapy scalp massage has been shown to effectively stimulate blood flow to the scalp and the underlying hair follicles to promote healthy hair growth. It is also helpful for stopping hair loss and hair thinning, both of which are of great concern for many modern day men and women.

Research conducted in Aberdeen, Scotland, by the Department of Dermatology showed successful outcomes for the use of essential oils in the treatment of alopecia. The results of the study showed aromatherapy massage to be a safe and effective treatment for alopecia areata. It also showed that treatment with essential oils was significantly more effective than treatment with a carrier oil alone.

In many ways, hair is similar to skin as it reflects your inner state of balance and health. A poor state of health can be responsible for dullness and loss of hair.

Men and women can suffer from age-related hair loss or thinning due to hormonal fluctuations during pregnancy and menopause. Research has shown that essential oils like palmarosa and geranium roseum and graveolens help to balance hormonal fluctuations that can lead to hair thinning and loss of hair.

Extreme stress can also play a significant role in hair loss for which the healing power of emotionally calming pure essential oils like clary sage, ylang ylang and German chamomile are highly recommended.

Most hair loss problems not directly caused by imbalances of health can usually be traced to maltreatment of the hair with excessive heat or chemical treatments like coloring and perming or washing with strong detergent-based shampoos.

These are the major causes of hair loss and can lead to dandruff and other common hair problems.

Hair and Scalp Treatment Program

Use either the "Stop Hair Loss Formula" (page 115) as a ready-to-use leave-on conditioner or the Scalp Reconditioning Formula below as an aromatherapy scalp massage daily for 10–14 days. Then, take a week long break before beginning the cycle of daily application for another 10–14 days.

Follow the instructions outlined and continue your application of either formula as needed to promote restoration of your hair's natural beauty, luster and health. Experiment with both formulas to find out which formula and application works best for getting the results you desire.

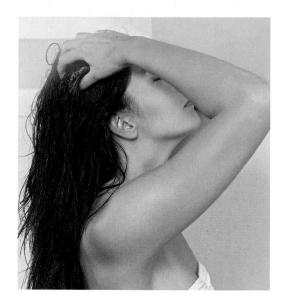

You can also add 1–2 drops of your Scalp Reconditioning Formula to your favorite carrier oil and use as a leave-on conditioner for up to an hour. Then shampoo your hair thoroughly afterward. Refer to the "Hair and Scalp Treatment Program" section for more about how to use your Scalp Reconditioning Formula.

Use this formula as an invigorating scalp massage oil to stop hair loss and to stimulate new hair growth. Apply daily for an invigorating scalp aromatherapy massage and leave on for about 1 hour. Shampoo thoroughly afterward.

Tip: To easily remove oil from the hair shaft, use your favorite shampoo (without the addition of water) to wash your hair. The shampoo will absorb the oil from the hair shaft. Then re-rinse the hair with warm water. Repeat if needed.

Scalp Reconditioning Formula

The Scalp Reconditioning Formula contains essential oils with stimulating, restorative and hormone-balancing properties known to be effective for stimulating new, healthy hair growth, as well as helping to stop hair loss and hair thinning.

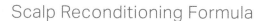

To a 5-ml, colored-glass, euro-dropper bottle add:

Vetiver: 30 drops

Ylang Ylang: 30 drops

Geranium Roseum and Graveolens: 15 drops each

Rosemary: 5 drops

Carrot Seed: 5 drops

Cap the bottle tightly and shake vigorously to blend the oils together. Allow to synergize for 24 hours or longer before using.

Scalp Massage Oil

Use the Scalp Reconditioning Formula as an invigorating scalp massage oil to stimulate new, healthy hair growth, or use the formula below.

To a 5-ml, colored-glass, euro-dropper bottle add:

Cypress: 20 drops

Lemon: 20 drops

Helichrysum: 40 drops

Birch: 10 drops

Juniper Berry: 10 drops

Close the cap tightly and shake the bottle vigorously to thoroughly blend the essential oils. Allow to synergize for 8 or more hours before using.

You can add 1–2 drops of your Scalp Massage Oil to your favorite carrier oil and use as a leave-in conditioner for up to an hour. Then shampoo your hair thoroughly after.

Stop Hair Loss (Alopecia) Formula

To stimulate new hair growth and to prevent or stop hair loss and hair thinning use this stimulating and restorative Stop Hair Loss Formula made of pure essential oils. The essential oils in this formula are known to be helpful for relieving stress and promoting hormone balance, which studies show can be contributing factors in hair loss.

To a 5-ml, colored-glass, euro-dropper bottle, add:

Blue Yarrow: 20 drops

Ylang Ylang: 20 drops

Palmarosa: 30 drops

Clary Sage: 10 drops

Cedarwood: 10 drops

Thyme: 5 drops

Rosemary Verbenone: 5 drops

(continued)

Stop Hair Loss (Alopecia)

Hair loss, hair thinning or baldness are a great concern for many people. The medical term for hair loss is alopecia, and it can be either partial (*alopecia areata*) or total (*alopecia totalis*).

There is often a great deal of psychological and emotional stress caused by one's appearance, especially in regards to hair loss. As hair plays a large role in one's overall identity, especially for women, hair loss can be an especially sensitive issue to talk about and is often experienced as a feeling of loss of control, loss of youth and even a loss of status in the world. Hair loss can lead to feelings of low self-esteem and can result in isolation from others. For cancer patients undergoing chemotherapy treatment, hair loss has been reported to forever change one's self-image and sense of belonging in the world.

A study on male pattern baldness compared Minoxidil (an over-the-counter hair loss product) to rosemary essential oil—just one of the ingredients in the Stop Hair Loss Formula. Groups rubbed either rosemary oil or Minoxidil into the scalp daily. At six months, both groups experienced a significant increase in hair growth, with rosemary users having less itchy scalps.

Cap the bottle tightly and shake vigorously to blend the oils together. Allow to synergize for 24 hours before using.

The simplest way to use your Stop Hair Loss Formula is to add 1–2 drops of it to your favorite shampoo. Use it as your regular hair wash to stimulate new, healthy hair growth and to prevent hair loss and thinning.

To make a ready-to-use Stop Hair Loss Formula, simply add 15 drops of your synergy blend to a 1-ounce (30-ml) bottle of your favorite carrier oil. Shake the bottle well to disperse the oils thoroughly. Apply enough of your formula to cover your scalp and saturate your hair shaft. Leave on for up to an hour to allow the oils time to be completely absorbed into your scalp and hair follicles. Shampoo your hair thoroughly afterward to completely remove the oil from your hair and scalp. Refer to the "Hair and Scalp Treatment Program" section on page 114 for more information about using essential oils to stop hair loss.

CAUTION: Please keep oils away from eyes, and do not apply oil directly on any open sores as this can cause sensitization to essential oils.

Lip Balms

Lip balm is excellent for moisturizing and healing dry, cracked and chapped lips often caused by environmental and weather conditions or simple dehydration. The waxy substance of lip balm applied topically over your lips effectively moisturizes them, as well as sealing and protecting them from exposure to harsh environments. The first lip balm may have been inspired by Lydia Maria Child's popular book, *The American Frugal Housewife*, in which Child recommended the use of an "earwax remedy successful when others have failed."

Dry, Chapped Lips Formula

Easy to make, this lip balm can be stored for long periods of time, a year or more when using vitamin E oil as a natural preservative and when sealed properly and stored in the refrigerator. Use it to heal dry, cracked or chapped lips and to smooth mouth wrinkles and prevent and treat cold sore outbreaks. An intensive, long-wear lip balm, this formula is non-greasy and petroleum-free. Formulated to moisturize and heal your lips, this lip balm makes a wonderful gift for friends and family members.

To a 5-ml, colored-glass, euro-dropper bottle add:
Lavender: 30 drops
Sandalwood: 50 drops
Ylang Ylang: 20 drops

Makes 8–10 (⅛-ounce [4-ml]) lip balm containers:
1 heaping tbsp (22 g) beeswax (Less makes your lip balm softer; more beeswax makes it more firm.)
¼ cup (60 ml) light coconut oil

Close cap tightly and shake bottle vigorously to thoroughly blend essential oils. Allow to synergize for 8 or more hours before using.

Put the beeswax and light coconut oil into a double boiler. For a homemade double boiler, use a glass measuring cup (such as Pyrex) inside a pan of water. Heat the mixture over medium-low heat until the beeswax melts.

Remove from the heat source and allow the liquid to cool slightly before adding your essential oils. Gently blend in the essential oils with a sterile instrument. Immediately pour the mixture into your lip balm containers and refrigerate to cool.

Apply liberally to your lips with your fingertips. Use as frequently as you like.

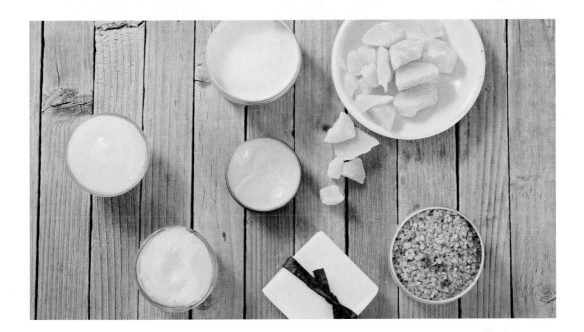

Severely Dry, Cracked, Chapped Lips Formula

The oils in this formula are known for their ability to regulate and heal dry, cracked and chapped lips.

To a 5-ml, colored-glass, euro-dropper bottle add:
Myrrh: 50 drops
Patchouli: 30 drops
Helichrysum: 20 drops

Cap tightly and shake bottle vigorously to thoroughly blend essential oils. Allow to synergize for 8 hours or more before using.

PLEASE NOTE: This is just one of the lip balm formulas, and directions for how to make lip balm are at the bottom of the the Dry, Chapped Lips Formula on page 116.

Cold Sore Formula

This Cold Sore Formula makes an intensive, long-wear lip balm, and is formulated with some of the most potent pure essential oils. These oils are beneficial for promoting fast relief and rapid healing of herpes simplex and cold sore outbreaks, and may help build your natural immunity against future outbreaks.

To a 5-ml, colored-glass, euro-dropper bottle add:
Tea Tree: 20 drops
Ravensara: 30 drops
Palmarosa: 50 drops

Makes 8–10 (⅛-ounce [4-ml]) lip balm containers:
1 heaping tbsp (22 g) beeswax (Less makes your lip balm softer; more beeswax makes it more firm.)
¼ cup (60 ml) light coconut oil

(continued)

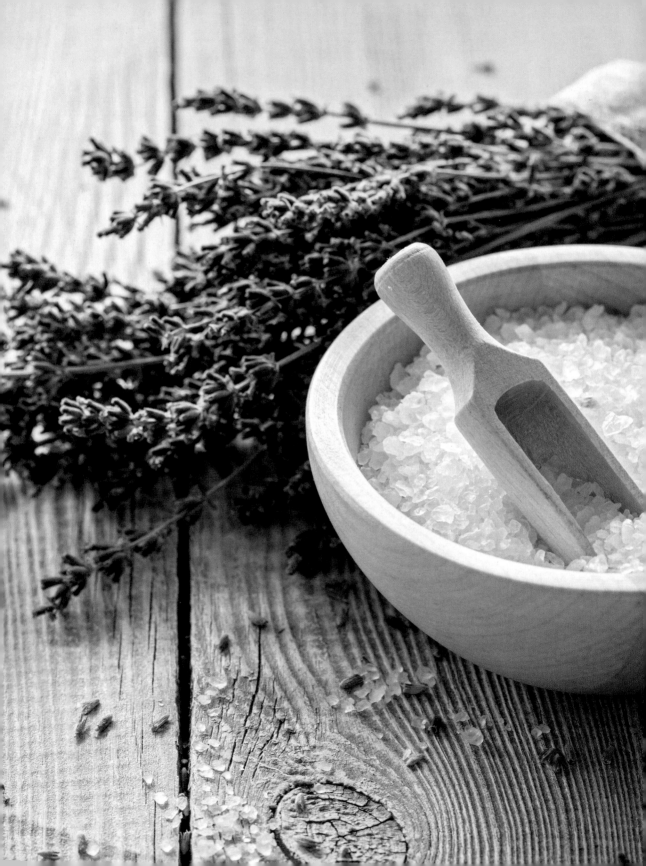

Close the cap tightly and shake the bottle vigorously to thoroughly blend the essential oils. Allow to synergize for 8 or more hours before using.

Put the beeswax and light coconut oil into a double boiler. For a homemade double boiler, use a glass measuring cup (such as Pyrex) inside a pan of water. Heat the mixture over medium-low heat until the beeswax melts.

Remove from the heat source and allow the liquid to cool slightly before adding your essential oils. Gently blend in the essential oils with a sterile instrument. Immediately pour the mixture into your lip balm containers and refrigerate to cool.

Apply liberally to your lips with your fingertips. Use as frequently as you like; it won't build up!

Exfoliating Sugar Scrubs

This natural exfoliating treatment is quick and easy to make. You can use a single essential oil in your sugar scrub, which is recommended if you have sensitive or problem skin. You can also use a blend of oils when you wish to achieve a broader spectrum of application and benefits. Use your sugar scrub before your bath or shower.

Exfoliating Sugar Scrub Oil Formula

An invigorating experience that will renew body, mind and soul.

1 cup (200 g) cane sugar, fine grain (exfoliating pore polish)

Substitute: 1 cup (200 g) raw brown sugar (aggressive exfoliation)

1–4 tsp (5–20 ml) favorite carrier oil (rose hip, light coconut or jojoba recommended)

1 drop pure essential oil

In a small ceramic bowl, mix together the sugar and your chosen carrier oil until thoroughly blended. Add one drop of pure essential oil or blend to the mixture and blend thoroughly. Add more carrier oil as desired if you prefer a loose, wet action for your sugar scrub.

Stand over a large bath towel or on a non-slip bath mat inside your tub. You can also lie on a plastic spa sheet as you begin to apply the sugar scrub. Rub the skin gently, using upward sweeping strokes, starting at the toes and working upward to the abdomen. Then begin to stroke upward from the fingertips to the shoulders.

After finishing your extremities, begin rubbing the sugar scrub onto the front side of your torso and then the backside.

You can rinse off the sugar scrub in a warm and soothing shower or take a steaming hot bath afterward.

After the sugar scrub, your skin will feel silky smooth and will have the appearance of being lustrous and more youthful!

pH Balancing Honey Lemon Sugar Facial Scrub Formula

One's pH balance is the key to having great skin. The letters pH stand for "potential hydrogen" and refer to the ratio of acid to alkaline balance of your body and skin. This ranges from 1 (most acidic) to 14 (most alkaline). A pH imbalance is the cause for almost every skin problem or issue, from acne to premature aging and wrinkling. There is a simple and easy fix for balancing your skin's pH, and it's the Honey Lemon Sugar Facial Scrub. According to dermatologist Patricia Wexler, MD, "The skin's barrier, which is known as the acid mantle, is responsible for keeping in lipids and moisture while blocking germs, pollution, toxins and bacteria.

(continued)

To work its best, the acid mantle should be slightly acidic, at a 5.5 pH balance. When it's too alkaline, skin becomes dry and sensitive; you may even get eczema. You may also experience inflammation, which inhibits the skin's ability to ward off matrix metalloproteinases [MMPs], the enzymes that destroy collagen and cause wrinkles and sagging."

This lovely mixture of honey, sugar, coconut oil and lemon pure essential oil will gently exfoliate your skin while balancing your skin's pH, leaving it feeling soft and silky smooth. It will also restore the skin's natural luster and shine. Lemon pure essential oil boosts the cleansing and skin tonic effects of this facial scrub. It's also a delightfully aromatic spa treatment for the brain as it relieves confusion and brings clarity, as well as calms anxiety and stress.

½ cup (100 g) sugar (raw brown or white)

½ cup (118 ml) light coconut oil (or favorite carrier oil)

4 tbsp (60 ml) raw honey

4 tsp (20 ml) lemon juice (fresh squeezed)

1 drop lemon pure essential oil

In a small ceramic bowl, blend the sugar and coconut oil (or other carrier oil). Then add honey, blending the mixture thoroughly together. Finally, add the fresh-squeezed lemon juice and lemon essential oil to the mixture and blend thoroughly.

With your fingertips, slowly and gently begin to apply the honey and lemon exfoliating scrub to your facial skin and polish the skin with it, making small, gentle circular movements. Begin at your décolletage and move upward, being sure to exfoliate your entire face, from the chin, over both cheeks and to the nose and forehead.

Be sure to use light, even pressure (10–60 seconds in each area) in small circular movements (clockwise and counter-clockwise) to remove old skin cells and cellular debris.

Rinse your face thoroughly with lukewarm water after you're done. Facial skin will feel invigorated and renewed and have a more youthful and radiant glow.

After your pH Balancing Honey Lemon Sugar Facial Scrub, drink plenty of pure, fresh water. You may wish to infuse your water with lemon pure essential oil diluted in a natural sweetener like stevia, honey or maple syrup. Drinking this throughout the day after your sugar scrub will help to keep your skin hydrated, your energy and stamina humming and your intellect switched on.

Salt Glow Treatments

A Salt Glow Treatment is an invigorating massage experience and is made with either sea salts or Epsom salts. This is one of the most inexpensive spa treatments you can use for deep exfoliation. Salt Glow Treatments renew and freshen your skin cell tissue and take only minutes to do, making them very easy to integrate into a busy and hectic lifestyle. Exfoliation is known to enhance circulation, as well as promote detoxification.

Each nourishing treatment is made with the pure essential oils known for balancing a particular skin type or condition, and all have the ability to freshen, tone and renew skin cell tissue. Use the following essential oil formulas by skin type or for balancing and healing a particular skin condition as noted.

Skin Healing and Regeneration Formula

If you tend to get blemishes frequently or have an uneven complexion, this is the formula for you.

To a 5-ml, colored-glass, euro-dropper bottle add:

Carrot Seed: 40 drops

Geranium Roseum and Graveolens: 20 drops each

Helichrysum: 20 drops

1 cup (500 g) Celtic (fine grind) or regular sea salt (detoxifier)

1–4 tsp (5–20 ml) favorite carrier oil (light coconut oil, jojoba or rose hip recommended)

Close the cap tightly and shake the bottle vigorously to thoroughly blend the essential oils. Allow to synergize for 8 or more hours before using.

Add the salt and carrier oil to a bowl, and then blend together until thoroughly mixed. Add 1–3 drops of the oil blend to the mixture and blend thoroughly. Add more carrier oil if you prefer a looser, more wet action for your salt glow.

Stand over a large bath towel or on a non-slip bath mat. Begin to apply your salt glow. Rub your skin gently using upward sweeping strokes. Start at your toes and work upward to your abdomen. Then begin to stroke upward from your fingertips to your shoulders.

After finishing your extremities, begin rubbing your salt glow onto the front side of your torso and then your backside. Use gentle circular movements on your upper torso, including your abdomen, chest, buttocks, backside and upper thighs.

After gently massaging your entire upper torso with the salt glow, you can rinse off in a warm and soothing shower. You can also relax in a steaming hot bath, steam room or sauna afterward. The salt glow will leave your skin feeling soft, supple and silky smooth, with a youthful appearance.

Regulating All Skin Types Formula

This is the best all-around salt glow formula to use for any skin type. It's a great place to start if you've never experienced a salt glow.

To a 5-ml, colored-glass, euro-dropper bottle add:

Geranium Bourbon: 40 drops

Carrot Seed: 20 drops

Ylang Ylang: 20 drops

Lavender: 20 drops

1 cup (500 g) Celtic (fine grind) or regular sea salt (detoxifier)

1–4 tsp (5–20 ml) favorite carrier oil (light coconut oil, jojoba or rose hip recommended)

Close the cap tightly and shake the bottle vigorously to thoroughly blend the essential oils. Allow to synergize for 8 or more hours before using.

Add the salt and carrier oil to a bowl, and then blend together until thoroughly mixed. Add 1–3 drops of the oil blend to the mixture and blend thoroughly. Add more carrier oil if you prefer a looser, more wet action for your salt glow.

Stand over a large bath towel or on a non-slip bath mat. Begin to apply your salt glow. Rub your skin gently using upward sweeping strokes. Start at your toes and work upward to your abdomen.

(continued)

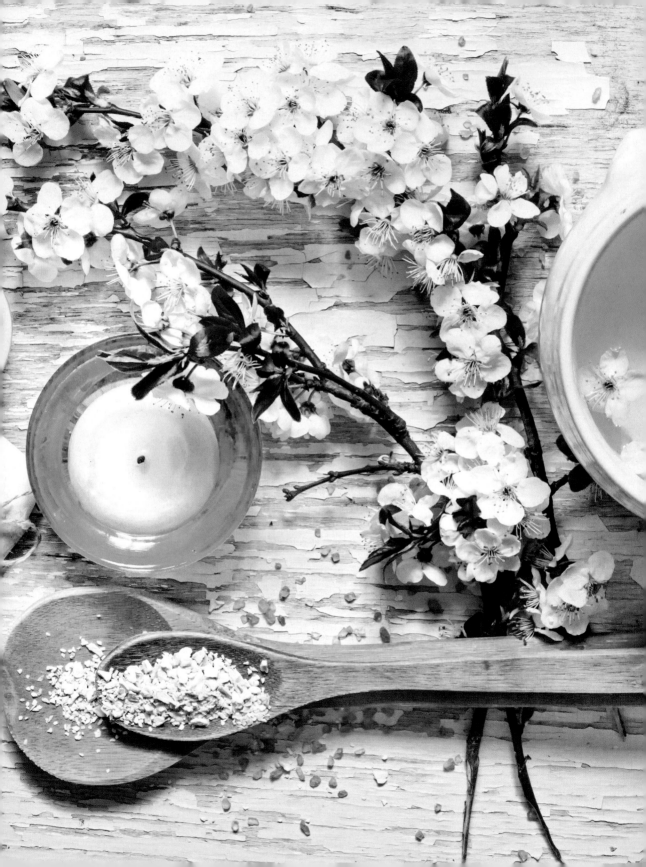

Then begin to stroke upward from your fingertips to your shoulders.

After finishing your extremitles, begin rubbing your salt glow onto the front side of your torso and then your backside. Use gentle circular movements on your upper torso, including your abdomen, chest, buttocks, backside and upper thighs.

After gently massaging your entire upper torso with the salt glow, you can rinse off in a warm and soothing shower. You can also relax in a steaming hot bath, steam room or sauna afterward.

The salt glow will leave your skin feeling soft, supple and silky smooth, with a youthful appearance.

PLEASE NOTE: Essential oils are not water-soluble, and you must use a dispersant when adding them to a bath. The water may cause the oils to penetrate your system more quickly or cause irritation to sensitive or damaged skin (such as open wounds, blemishes, sores or rashes).

Chronic Skin Conditions Formula

If you have a chronic skin condition (such as eczema, rosacea, rash, dermatitis or psoriasis), this is the best skin formula to use to bring balance and harmony to skin cell tissue.

To a 5-ml, colored-glass, euro-dropper bottle add:
Palmarosa: 40 drops
German Chamomile: 20 drops
Helichrysum: 20 drops
Spikenard: 20 drops

1 cup (500 g) Celtic (fine grind) or regular sea salt (detoxifier)
1–4 tsp (5–20 ml) favorite carrier oil (light coconut oil, jojoba or rose hip recommended)

Close the cap tightly and shake the bottle vigorously to thoroughly blend the essential oils. Allow to synergize for 8 or more hours before using

Add salt and carrier oil to a bowl, and then blend together until thoroughly mixed. Add 1–3 drops of the oil blend to the mixture and blend thoroughly. Add more carrier oil if you prefer a looser, more wet action for your salt glow.

Stand over a large bath towel or on a non-slip bath mat. Begin to apply your salt glow. Rub your skin gently using upward sweeping strokes. Start at your toes and work upward to your abdomen.

Then begin to stroke upward from your fingertips to your shoulders.

After finishing your extremities, begin rubbing your salt glow onto the front side of your torso and then your backside. Use gentle circular movements on your upper torso, including your abdomen, chest, buttocks, backside and upper thighs.

After gently massaging your entire upper torso with the salt glow, you can rinse off in a warm and soothing shower. You can also relax in a steaming hot bath, steam room or sauna afterwards.

The salt glow will leave your skin feeling soft, supple and silky smooth, with a youthful appearance.

PLEASE NOTE: Essential oils are not water-soluble, and you must use a dispersant when adding them to a bath. The water may cause the oils to penetrate your system more quickly or cause irritation to sensitive or damaged skin (such as open wounds, blemishes, sores or rashes).

Regulating and Balancing, Wound Healing, Problem Skin Formula

If you have acne outbreaks, combination skin, problem skin or sensitive skin, this is the salt glow formula for you to use.

To a 5-ml, colored-glass, euro-dropper bottle add:

Blue Yarrow: 40 drops

Palmarosa: 40 drops

Helichrysum: 10 drops

Geranium Roseum and Graveolens: 5 drops each

1 cup (500 g) Celtic (fine grind) or regular sea salt (detoxifier)

1–4 tsp (5–20 ml) favorite carrier oil (light coconut oil, jojoba or rose hip recommended)

Close the cap tightly and shake the bottle vigorously to thoroughly blend the essential oils. Allow to synergize for 8 or more hours before using.

Add the salt and carrier oil to a bowl, and then blend together until thoroughly mixed. Add 1–3 drops of the oil blend to the mixture and blend thoroughly. Add more carrier oil if you prefer a looser, more wet action for your salt glow.

Stand over a large bath towel or on a non-slip bath mat. Begin to apply your salt glow. Rub your skin gently using upward sweeping strokes. Start at your toes and work upward to your abdomen.

Then begin to stroke upward from your fingertips to your shoulders.

After finishing your extremities, begin rubbing your salt glow onto the front side of your torso and then your backside. Use gentle circular movements on your upper torso, including your abdomen, chest, buttocks, backside and upper thighs.

After gently massaging your entire upper torso with the salt glow, you can rinse off in a warm and soothing shower. You can also relax in a steaming hot bath, steam room or sauna afterward.

The salt glow will leave your skin feeling soft, supple and silky smooth, with a youthful appearance.

PLEASE NOTE: Essential oils are not water-soluble, and you must use a dispersant when adding them to a bath. The water may cause the oils to penetrate your system more quickly or cause irritation to sensitive or damaged skin (such as open wounds, blemishes, sores or rashes).

Moisture Balancing and Healing for All Skin Types Formula

An ideal beauty formula for all skin types.

To a 5-ml, colored-glass, euro-dropper bottle add:

Spikenard: 40 drops

Lavender: 20 drops

Ylang Ylang III: 20 drops

Carrot Seed: 20 drops

1 cup (500 g) Celtic (fine grind) or regular sea salt (detoxifier)

1–4 tsp (5–20 ml) favorite carrier oil (light coconut oil, jojoba or rose hip recommended)

Close the cap tightly and shake the bottle vigorously to thoroughly blend the essential oils. Allow to synergize for 8 or more hours before using.

Add the salt and carrier oil to a bowl, and then blend together until thoroughly mixed. Add 1–3 drops of the oil blend to the mixture and blend thoroughly. Add more carrier oil if you prefer a looser, more wet action for your salt glow.

Stand over a large bath towel or on a non-slip bath mat. Begin to apply your salt glow. Rub your skin gently using upward sweeping strokes. Start at your toes and work upward to your abdomen.

Then begin to stroke upward from your finger-tips to your shoulders.

After finishing your extremities, begin rubbing your salt glow onto the front side of your torso and then your backside. Use gentle circular movements on your upper torso, including your abdomen, chest, buttocks, backside and upper thighs.

After gently massaging your entire upper torso with the salt glow, you can rinse off in a warm and soothing shower. You can also relax in a steaming hot bath, steam room or sauna afterward.

The salt glow will leave your skin feeling soft, supple and silky smooth, with a youthful appearance.

PLEASE NOTE: Essential oils are not water-soluble, and you must use a dispersant when adding them to a bath. The water may cause the oils to penetrate your system more quickly or cause irritation to sensitive or damaged skin (such as open wounds, blemishes, sores or rashes).

Oily Skin Formula

The essential oils in this formula are ideal for regulating and balancing oily skin types.

To a 5-ml, colored-glass, euro-dropper bottle add:
Cypress: 40 drops
Lemon: 20 drops
Palmarosa: 20 drops
Helichrysum: 10 drops
Geranium Rocoum and Graveolens: 5 drops each

1 cup (500 g) Celtic (fine grind) or regular sea salt (detoxifier)
1–4 tsp (5–20 ml) favorite carrier oil (light coconut oil, jojoba or rose hip recommended)

Close the cap tightly and shake the bottle vigorously to thoroughly blend the essential oils. Allow to synergize for 8 or more hours before using.

Add the salt and carrier oil to a bowl, and then blend together until thoroughly mixed. Add 1–3 drops of the oil blend to the mixture and blend thoroughly. Add more carrier oil if you prefer a looser, more wet action for your salt glow.

Stand over a large bath towel or on a non-slip bath mat. Begin to apply your salt glow. Rub your skin gently using upward sweeping strokes. Start at your toes and work upward to your abdomen.

Then begin to stroke upward from your finger-tips to your shoulders.

(continued)

After finishing your extremities, begin rubbing your salt glow onto the front side of your torso and then your backside. Use gentle circular movements on your upper torso, including your abdomen, chest, buttocks, backside and upper thighs.

After gently massaging your entire upper torso with the salt glow, you can rinse off in a warm and soothing shower. You can also relax in a steaming hot bath, steam room or sauna afterward.

The salt glow will leave your skin feeling soft, supple and silky smooth, with a youthful appearance.

PLEASE NOTE: Essential oils are not water-soluble, and you must use a dispersant when adding them to a bath. The water may cause the oils to penetrate your system more quickly or cause irritation to sensitive or damaged skin (such as open wounds, blemishes, sores or rashes).

Dry and Mature Skin Formula

The oils in this formula help regulate and moisturize dry and mature skin cells.

To a 5-ml, colored-glass, euro-dropper bottle add:
Palmarosa: 60 drops
Helichrysum: 20 drops
Geranium Roseum and Graveolens: 5 drops each
Rosemary Verbenone: 10 drops

1 cup (500 g) Celtic (fine grind) or regular sea salt (detoxifier)
1–4 tsp (5–20 ml) favorite carrier oil (light coconut oil, jojoba or rose hip recommended)

Close the cap tightly and shake the bottle vigorously to thoroughly blend the essential oils. Allow to synergize for 8 or more hours before using.

Add the salt and carrier oil to a bowl, and then blend together until thoroughly mixed. Add 1–3 drops of the oil blend to the mixture and blend thoroughly. Add more carrier oil if you prefer a looser, more wet action for your salt glow.

Stand over a large bath towel or on a non-slip bath mat. Begin to apply your salt glow. Rub your skin gently using upward sweeping strokes. Start at your toes and work upward to your abdomen.

Then begin to stroke upward from your fingertips to your shoulders.

After finishing your extremities, begin rubbing your salt glow onto the front side of your torso and then your backside. Use gentle circular movements on your upper torso, including your abdomen, chest, buttocks, backside and upper thighs.

After gently massaging your entire upper torso with the salt glow, you can rinse off in a warm and soothing shower. You can also relax in a steaming hot bath, steam room or sauna afterward.

The salt glow will leave your skin feeling soft, supple and silky smooth, with a youthful appearance.

PLEASE NOTE: Essential oils are not water-soluble, and you must use a dispersant when adding them to a bath. The water may cause the oils to penetrate your system more quickly or cause irritation to sensitive or damaged skin (such as open wounds, blemishes, sores or rashes).

Additional Body Treatments

Complete your spa treatments with a French Clay Body Mask and some Healing and Regenerative Body Butter (page 129) for the ultimate spa experience.

French Clay Body Mask Formula

This clay body mask made with French clay and pure essential oils will cleanse, detoxify and improve your skin's elasticity. Create a nice ambience for your French Clay Body Mask experience by turning off all phones and electronic devices. Make sure the room is comfortably warm, but not hot. Light a candle and play gentle and relaxing music in the background, or just relax and allow yourself to be silent during your treatment.

To a 5-ml, colored-glass, euro-dropper bottle add:

Lavender: 40 drops

Ylang Ylang III: 40 drops

Carrot Seed: 15 drops

Rosemary Verbenone: 5 drops

½–1½ cups (120–363 g) French pink or green clay* (partial or full body mask)
½–1½ cups (118–355 ml) purified water or cream (partial or full body mask)

1–4 drops French Clay Body Mask Formula

For a partial body mask: Add 1 drop of the essential oil blend to the clay

For a full body mask: Add 3–4 drops of the essential oil blend to the clay

*Clay can stain fabric so take care to use a plastic covering to prevent staining.

(continued)

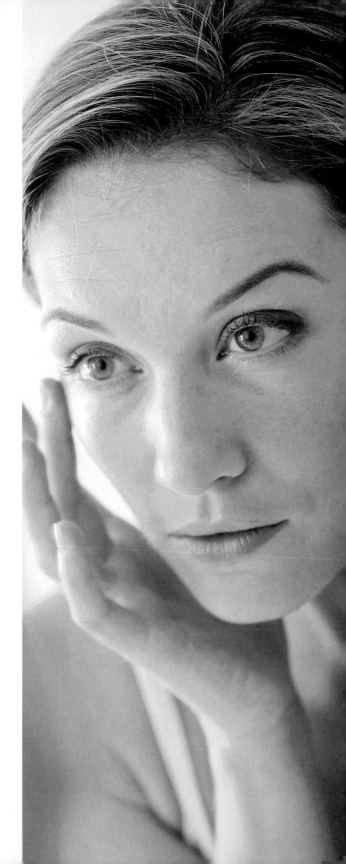

Close the cap tightly and shake the bottle vigorously to thoroughly blend the essential oils. Allow to synergize for 8 or more hours before using.

Add your choice of natural French clay to a bowl. Then begin to blend in purified water or cream to make a loose paste, but make sure it's not totally wet. When the clay paste is the desired wetness, add your essential oil blend and mix in thoroughly.

Stand over a large bath towel or on a slip-proof bath mat and immediately begin applying the French clay mixture to a body part or to the entire body using gentle, upward sweeping strokes.

After you've finished applying the clay mask, it's time to relax and allow the mask to dry. You can lie down in a dry tub and drape the large bath towel lightly over you if needed, so you don't get chilled. Or you can lie down on a large bath towel or plastic spa sheet and cover yourself lightly with another large bath towel. You want air to circulate around your skin, so the clay will dry and produce the drawing effect on your skin tissues to pull out toxins and exfoliate, but you don't want to get chilled either. The best way to do this is by making sure the room is comfortably warm before starting your treatment.

Allow the mask to dry for 10–20 minutes, and then rinse off in a warm shower. Towel dry with a soft towel. Wrap yourself in a snuggly robe and relax for 10–15 minutes afterward in a lounging chair, or lie down in your bed. Be sure to hydrate during and after your treatment by drinking pure, fresh water with a slice of lemon or lime.

Your skin will feel soft, refreshed and toned after the mask.

Healing and Regenerative Body Butter Formula

This healing and regenerative body butter made with pure essential oils is absolutely exquisite for balancing and nourishing your skin cell tissues. Use this youth-enhancing, healing and regenerative body butter as an anti-aging preventative treatment, as well as to smooth the appearance of deep lines and wrinkles.

Each of the recommended pure essential oils has a long history of use for skincare. Effective for renewing mature, aged or weathered skin and fading age spots, its notable balancing, moisturizing, rejuvenating and anti-inflammatory properties make it excellent for treating an assortment of skin issues.

Try the Healing and Regenerative Body Butter Formula for relieving these skin conditions:

- Rosacea
- Rash
- Acne
- Scars
- Blemishes
- Bruises
- Dermatitis
- Eczema
- Psoriasis
- Shingles
- Herpes

Recipe makes approximately 4 ounces (120 ml).

Use organic ingredients if available.

2 tbsp (27 g) pure shea and/or cocoa butter (moisturizer)

1 tbsp (14 g) beeswax

4 tbsp (60 ml) light fractionated coconut oil

1 tbsp (15 ml) vegetable glycerin (improves smoothness and lubrication)

60 drops sandalwood essential oil

60 drops helichrysum essential oil

60–90 drops one or more pure essential oils of your choice (lavender, ylang ylang, rose or geranium)

Optional: 4–6 drops vitamin E oil (natural preservative)

4-oz (120-ml), colored-glass jar with tight-fitting lid

Put shea or cocoa butter, or a combination of both, along with the beeswax, into the light fractionated coconut oil. Heat in a double boiler or in your homemade double boiler (a glass measuring cup inside a pan of water, over medium-low heat).

Heat this mixture until the shea and/or cocoa butter and beeswax are melted thoroughly together.

Remove the melted ingredients from the double boiler or take the glass measuring cup from the pan. Add vegetable glycerin and blend the mixture together with a sterile instrument.

After cooling the butter mixture slightly, add in your essential oil blend gently with a sterile instrument. Add the vitamin E oil, if desired.

Pour the butter into your colored-glass jar and allow to set completely before using. Seal tightly with a lid and store in a cool, dry place.

Body butter will keep for 6 months or longer if properly sealed and stored.

Healing Bath Salts Formula

Set the mood and ambience for a healing bath spa experience by making sure you are in a quiet space where you will not be disturbed for at least 45 minutes or longer. All phones and electronic devices should be turned off. Light a candle and play gentle and relaxing music in the background, or just relax and allow yourself to be silent.

This relaxing and rejuvenating Healing Bath Salts Formula is helpful for letting go of your cares and worries. It is soothing to an agitated state of mind. The essential oils are known for their sedative action and ability to promote inner balance, peace and calm, and are renewing to your chakra energy system.

To a 5-ml, colored-glass, euro-dropper bottle add:

Red Mandarin: 40 drops

Lavender: 10 drops

Ylang Ylang III: 20 drops

Clary Sage: 10 drops

Frankincense: 20 drops

1 cup (500 g) Epsom salts (muscle relaxant, detoxifier)

1 cup (275 g) Celtic (grey) salts (rich in minerals)

1 cup (520 g) baking soda (skin softener)

Optional ingredient: ½ cup (115 g) green or pink clay

5–12 drops Healing Bath Salts Formula

Close the cap tightly and shake the bottle vigorously to thoroughly blend the essential oils. Allow to synergize for 8 or more hours before using.

Blend together your Epsom and Celtic sea salts, baking soda and choice of clay, if desired, in a small ceramic bowl.

Add 5–12 drops of the Healing Bath Salts Formula to the salts and thoroughly blend the ingredients together.

Add 1–3 cups (500–1,500 g) of the scented bath salts mixture to your bathtub filled with warm water (preferably under 101°F [38°C]).

Soak for 20–30 minutes for a healing and rejuvenating bath spa experience.

After the soak, rinse off in a warm shower and towel dry. Then wrap yourself in a warm, snuggly robe and rest for 10–15 minutes in a comfortable lounging chair, or lie down for a nap in your bed.

Be sure to hydrate well during and after the bath. Water with fresh squeezed lemon or lime is perfect for revitalizing your adrenals and other organs.

Natural sea salts are rich in minerals and charged with electrical and healing properties that you can especially benefit from in a warm bath. A sea salt bath with pure essential oils is an effective way to cleanse and restore your chakras and auric energy field. You can purchase natural sea salt in your local health-food store in the spice section. For even more about baths, check out the "How to Use Essential Oils" section (page 20).

PLEASE NOTE: Essential oils are not water-soluble. You must use a dispersant when adding them to a bath. Water may cause the oils to penetrate your system more quickly or cause irritation to sensitive or damaged skin (such as blemishes, sores or rashes).

Around the *House*

Clear Stagnant Energy

We've all been in environments and around certain people or situations that afterward we can't seem to shake off their influence. It's like we've picked up "bad vibes," and they've stuck to us.

Quantum mechanics has now shown that negativity or bad vibes is a measure of quantum entanglement, which can easily be computed.

Since ancient times, energy medicine practitioners, natural healers and shamans from around the world have been practicing energy clearing techniques. Plant aromatics have a long history of use for this purpose. The scent of plant aromatics has been used effectively to clear negative and stagnant energy from a house or room, as well from the auric field of a person.

The essential oils traditionally used and recommended for clearing negative energy all have highly astringent properties, which when used on surface objects are known to break down sticky substances like gum, built up dirt and stubborn grime. The oils recommended for energy clearing also have a powerfully refreshing and restorative effect on the mind and emotions, as well as strong antimicrobial action.

Energy Clearing Formula

Use to clean floors, walls and all surfaces and countertops, as well as to clear and freshen the atmosphere of a room. You can also use the energy clearing formula to clear the aura or energy field of a person.

To a 5-ml, colored-glass, euro-dropper bottle add:

Lemon: 20 drops

Peppermint: 20 drops

Cypress: 20 drops

Cinnamon Leaf: 20 drops

Frankincense: 5 drops

Myrrh: 5 drops

Black Pepper: 5 drops

Juniper Berry: 5 drops

Close the cap tightly and shake the bottle vigorously to thoroughly blend the essential oils. Allow to synergize for 8 or more hours before using.

This formula is effective when diffused into the air or used as an aromatic room mist. For general, all-purpose cleaning, dilute the Energy Clearing Formula blend in warm soapy water to clean floors and walls, shampoo rugs and clean surfaces and countertops. This formula will also clear and freshen the atmosphere of a room. Be especially mindful to clean any darkened corners and thresholds. Dispose of dirty cleaning waters down a toilet.

To make a ready-to-use blend that you can wear as a perfume oil blend, simply add 15–30 drops of your synergy blend to a 1-ounce (30-ml) bottle of your favorite carrier oil. Shake the bottle well to disperse the oils thoroughly. Apply a few drops of your ready-to-use blend to your heart area, sinus points around your nose and forehead, as well as on the back of your neck and behind both ears.

Eliminate Odors

The synthetic fragrance industry is a booming business. Most of the fragrances available on the world market simply mask odors, but do not actually eliminate them. Additionally, petroleum-based fragrances can cause reactions and are thought to result in the development of allergies.

However, essential oils, unlike synthetic fragrances, are not only natural substances, but they seldom cause reactions or sensitization when used properly.

Essential oils are chemical chelators. They make chemicals nontoxic by fracturing their molecular structure. European scientists have found that essential oils work as natural chelators, bonding to metals and chemicals and ferrying them out of the body. In this same way they act to break down and eliminate odors.

This same ability to fracture molecular structure gives essential oils the ability to break down odor molecules and eliminate odors completely.

Deodorizer Formula

For odor-free air that is also pollution-free and safe to breathe, use the Deodorizer Formula. Essential oils can deodorize stale and bad odors caused by mold and mildew, smoke, skunk, rotten eggs, food, the garbage can, compost and foot and body odor, just to name a few.

To a 5-ml, colored-glass, euro-dropper bottle add:
Black Spruce: 30 drops
Lemon: 20 drops
Cinnamon Leaf: 20 drops
Peppermint: 20 drops
Cypress: 10 drops

Close the cap tightly and shake the bottle vigorously to thoroughly blend the essential oils. Allow to synergize for 8 or more hours before using.

This formula is effective when diffused into the air or used as an aromatic room mist. For general, all-purpose deodorizing, add the deodorizer blend to warm soapy water and use to clean floors and walls, shampoo rugs and clean surfaces and countertops. This formula will also deodorize, clear and freshen the atmosphere of a room. Be especially mindful to clean any darkened corners and thresholds. Dispose of dirty cleaning waters down a toilet.

To make a simple cleaner, add the deodorizer blend to either white vinegar or baking soda and use as an air freshener in your refrigerator and underneath sinks to effectively remove odors.

Air Freshener

Because of their ability to fracture the molecular structure of chemicals, essential oils are highly prized in the air freshener industry. Removing the source or cause of an offensive aroma is, of course, preferable to masking it from human perception for brief periods of time.

Like a breath of fresh air, essential oils will help you maintain the indoor air quality of your home and quickly eliminate unpleasant and unwanted odors.

Air Freshener Formula

Use to freshen a stale room, eliminate odors in areas with poor ventilation and enhance the ambience of any room with odor-free air that is also pollution-free and safe to breathe.

To a 5-ml, colored-glass, euro-dropper bottle add:
Lemongrass: 40 drops
Lemon: 20 drops
Peppermint: 20 drops
Cypress: 10 drops
Cinnamon Leaf: 10 drops
Black Spruce: 1–5 drops

Close the cap tightly and shake the bottle vigorously to thoroughly blend the essential oils. Allow to synergize for 8 or more hours before using.

This formula is effective when diffused into the air or used as an aromatic room mist. To make a simple cleaner, add the Air Freshener Formula to either white vinegar or baking soda and use as an air freshener in your refrigerator and underneath sinks to effectively remove odors.

Laundry Care

Personal hygiene is the foundation of your health, which is easily your most valuable asset. A high standard of cleaning and laundry care for all of your clothing and linens gives you the added protection and support needed in today's toxic world that is filled with harsh chemicals and pollutants. Use essential oils in your laundry to keep your health robust and to stay well and happy year-round.

Washer Formula

This formula is suitable for all your washing needs to freshen and sanitize.

To a 5-ml, colored-glass, euro-dropper bottle add:
Lemon: 50 drops
Peppermint: 20 drops
Eucalyptus: 20 drops
Oregano: 10 drops

Close the cap tightly and shake the bottle vigorously to thoroughly blend the essential oils. Allow to synergize for 8 or more hours before using.

Add 3–4 drops of the Washer Formula blend to your laundry detergent at the start of your washing cycle. For those who are allergic to dust mites, eucalyptus globulus may kill dust mites in bedding.

PLEASE NOTE: Excessive use of essential oils in your washer may damage plastic or hard rubber parts.

Dryer Formula

Leaves your clothes and linens smelling fresh and like new.

To a 5-ml, colored-glass, euro-dropper bottle add:
Lavender: 50 drops
Lemon: 30 drops
Peppermint: 20 drops

Close the cap tightly and shake the bottle vigorously to thoroughly blend the essential oils. Allow to synergize for 8 or more hours before using.

Add 3–4 drops of the dryer blend to a cotton cloth or pad and place in your dryer during the cool down, air fluff or wrinkle release cycle. Lavender oil will give your bedding and towels a clean, fresh scent and promote relaxation and calm, while lemon and peppermint remove greasy and oily smells and grime from your laundry.

Eco-Friendly Cleaning Supplies

Adding essential oils known for their antibacterial and antiviral powers to your dishpan or scrub bucket will kill germs and leave your home and living environments smelling clean and fresh. Eco-friendly cleaning supplies made with pure essential oils also have the added benefit of eliminating odors for pollution-free air that is safer to breathe.

All-Purpose Household Surface Cleaner Formula

Use to clean all surfaces and countertops of grease and grime and to remove oily stains, sticky substances, grime and dirty residue.

To a 5-ml, colored-glass, euro-dropper bottle add:
Lemon: 40 drops
Peppermint: 20 drops
Cypress: 20 drops
Black Pepper: 10 drops
Juniper Berry: 10 drops

Close the cap tightly and shake the bottle vigorously to thoroughly blend the essential oils. Allow to synergize for 8 or more hours before using.

For use as a powerful, general, all-purpose household cleaner, dilute 4–8 drops of the surface cleaner blend in a dishpan or sink filled with warm soapy water and use to clean all surfaces. Wipe down kitchen counters and bathroom surfaces with these cleansing, germicidal oils.

Dish Wash Formula

Use to wash your dishes, to cut grease and remove built-up grime, oily stains, sticky substances and dirty residue.

To a 5-ml, colored-glass, euro-dropper bottle add:

Lemon: 40 drops

Lavender: 20 drops

Cypress: 20 drops

Tea Tree: 20 drops

Close the cap tightly and shake the bottle vigorously to thoroughly blend the essential oils. Allow to synergize for 8 or more hours before using.

For use as a powerful dish-washing and all-purpose cleansing and germicidal agent, dilute 4–8 drops of the dish wash blend in a dishpan or sink filled with warm soapy water. Use to wash dishes and as a general, all-purpose cleanser. This formula is also great for cleaning stubborn and burnt food particles from pots and pans.

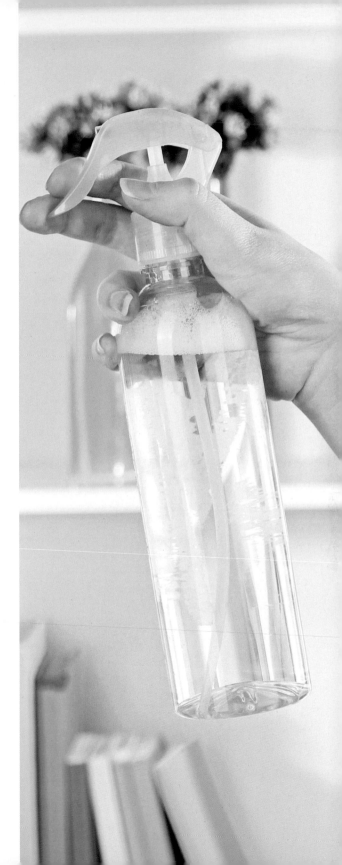

CHAPTER 13

Essential Oils in the
Workplace and Daily Life

Introducing Essential Oils into Your Professional Practice, Home or Workplace

When introducing pure essential oils and aromatherapy into your daily life—whether at home, in your professional practice or in your workplace—always remember that less is more. Pure essential oils are extremely concentrated; one drop of pure essential oil is generally equal to 3–4 cups (121–161 g) of plant matter. Even a drop or two can produce significant and immediate results upon inhalation or application.

Slowly introduce your oils, whether using them for yourself or with others, and observe the response to a single essential oil first before introducing more complex aromatherapy blends.

Listen to and watch for signs of sensitivity or displeasure for a particular scent. An essential oil may have the chemical constituents to produce the desired results, but its aroma may not be well tolerated. Remember the greatest benefits of aromatherapy can be enjoyed simply through inhaling their aroma, so it's essential to choose oils that are enjoyed for their aromatic scent, as well as the benefits of their chemical properties.

As the nose becomes accustomed to a wide spectrum of aromas for enjoyment, the response to different essential oils will change over time. When you are first learning, it's advisable to keep notes in your aromatherapy journal about how you, or someone you are administering essential oils to, are responding and being affected. This will help to expand your knowledge about aromatherapy and discover the best methods of application for obtaining consistently good results in practice. Through keeping an aromatherapy journal you will also develop your intuition for which aromas or blends to use when treating a wide variety of conditions.

Improve Productivity

Productivity, whether at home or work, is a major concern for most of us. We want to make the best and most efficient use of our time to achieve the things we value most and our top priorities in life. Whether you're a student completing a homework assignment or project, a busy mom caring for your home and family or an executive managing hundreds of employees, the need to be productive is of great importance to you. Productivity is always connected with achieving your bottom line, whatever that might be for you.

Research has shown essential oils help to increase productivity by as much as 54 percent when diffused into the workroom. There are many courses available, and corporations spend thousands of dollars to learn how to become more productive. Essential oils can help you become more productive just by inhaling their scent for a nominal cost.

Improve Productivity Formula

This may be the perfect solution when you need help focusing for prolonged periods on work projects, homework, arts and crafts and various daily routines. Use this blend of stimulating essential oils when you need to focus on a task with your complete attention, as well as to aid memory retention. This formula may also be helpful for children diagnosed with ADD.

To a 5-ml, colored-glass, euro-dropper bottle add:

Peppermint: 50 drops

Lemon: 20 drops

Cinnamon Leaf: 20 drops

Basil: 1–3 drops

Rosemary Verbenone: 1–3 drops

Black Spruce: 1–3 drops

Atlas Cedarwood: 10 drops

Close the cap tightly and shake the bottle vigorously to thoroughly blend the essential oils. Allow to synergize for 8 or more hours before using.

Dispense 1–3 drops on a cotton ball or smell strip and inhale the aromatic vapors of your Improve Productivity Formula blend for 10–15 seconds. You may repeat as needed. This blend may also be effective as an aromatic mist.

To make a ready-to-use Improve Productivity Formula blend that you can wear like a perfume oil, simply add 15–30 drops of your synergy blend to a 1-ounce (30-ml) bottle of your favorite carrier oil. Shake the bottle well to disperse the oils thoroughly. Apply a few drops of your ready-to-use blend to sinus points around your nose and forehead, as well as on the back of your neck.

Stimulate Curiosity and Creativity

As children, we seem to have an infinite capacity for being creative and curious about everything. Your favorite word as a child may have been "why." Your "why" is at the heart of taking action to do anything. "Why" is the motivating factor that connects you with the enthusiasm needed for doing anything in life. Find a big enough "why" and you will persevere to overcome any obstacle on the way to accomplishing your goal. If you want to create change in your life circumstances, it is very important that you ask new questions to get different results. In other words, you must be curious about what's not working in your life to begin to see patterns at work that you need to change to get different results. If you keep doing what you've been doing, you'll keep getting the same results. That's great if you are 100 percent happy with your results in life; however, most of us are not.

Another key question to ask when increasing your capacity for creativity and curiosity is the question, "What else could this mean?" Motivation expert Tony Robbins, a master of creating transformation and change, reminds us to ask the question "What else could this mean?" continually. Research has now shown that we don't see the world as it is, but as we are. We filter out anything that is happening that does not fit into our belief system. So, there you have two of the most important questions to begin asking when working to increase your capacity for curiosity and creativity and to make changes for the better in your life.

Stimulate Curiosity and Creativity Formula

This formula helps to renew your creative drive.

To a 5-ml, colored-glass, euro-dropper bottle add:

Grapefruit: 20 drops

Lemongrass: 40 drops

Palmarosa: 10 drops

Cinnamon Leaf: 10 drops

Spikenard: 10 drops

Frankincense: 10 drops

Black Pepper: 1–3 drops

Close the cap tightly and shake the bottle vigorously to thoroughly blend the essential oils. Allow to synergize for 8 or more hours before using.

Dispense 1–3 drops on a cotton ball or smell strip and inhale the aromatic vapors of your Stimulate Curiosity and Creativity Formula blend for 10–15 seconds. You may repeat as needed. This blend may also be effective as an aromatic mist.

To make a ready-to-use blend you can wear like a perfume oil, simply add 15–30 drops of your synergy blend to a 1-ounce (30-ml) bottle of your favorite carrier oil. Shake the bottle well to disperse the oils thoroughly. Apply a few drops of your ready-to-use blend to sinus points around your nose and forehead, as well as on the back of your neck.

Focus Support and Pay Attention Formula

Essential oils can help you to develop your ability to control the focus of your attention and shift into a positive emotional state at will.

Most educators and psychologists agree that your ability to focus on a task without distraction and pay attention is absolutely essential for achieving your goals.

A study conducted on 232 pairs of twins showed there was a direct correlation between temperament (frequency and intensity of temper tantrums, crying, moodiness and demanding attention) and attention span. The study showed that the twin with the most ability for absorption of an activity was much less temperamental.

Another study of 2,600 children also showed that "early exposure to television (around age two) was associated with later attention issues such as impulsiveness, disorganization and distractibility at age seven."

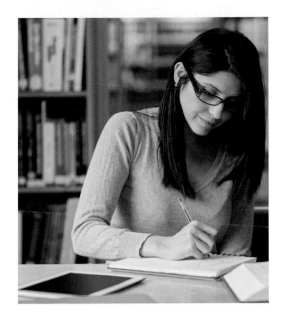

To a 5-ml, colored-glass, euro-dropper bottle add:

Peppermint: 40 drops

Rosemary: 1–2 drops

Lemon: 40 drops (or 80 drops if you don't want to use peppermint in your recipe)

Basil: 1–2 drops

Cedarwood: 20 drops

Close the cap tightly and shake the bottle vigorously to thoroughly blend the essential oils. Allow to synergize for 8 or more hours before using.

Adult Directions

Dispense 1–3 drops on a smell strip, cotton ball or tissue and inhale.

This blend may also be used in a diffuser and diffused into a room.

Use your Focus Support and Pay Attention Formula as needed for focus support, to pay attention and to stay alert naturally.

Children Directions

Allow children to self-select the oils to use alone or in a synergy blend. Pure essential oils may be too strong for their sensitive nervous systems, and you may wish to dilute the oils to 1–10 percent in a vegetable carrier oil like pure fractionated coconut oil.

CAUTION: Research indicates that peppermint oil may aggravate GERD (gastro esophageal reflux disease), a type of heartburn. Due to its strong cooling action, peppermint should not be used by children under two and a half years of age.

Essential Oils: Quick Reference Guides

Safety and Dilution Guide

Below are sample dilution guidelines I use for my aromatherapy products.

Guide for Standard Dilution of Essential Oils in Carrier Oil

Adults (25+ years): 15 drops EO in 1 ounce (30 ml) of carrier oil

Children age eighteen and older: 10 drops EO in 1 ounce (30 ml) of carrier oil

Children age ten to eighteen: 6–9 drops EO in 1 ounce (30 ml) of carrier oil

Children age five to ten: 5 drops EO in 1 ounce (30 ml) of carrier oil

Children age four and the elderly and infirm: 4 drops EO in 1 ounce (30 ml) of carrier oil

Children age three: 3 drops EO in 1 ounce (30 ml) of carrier oil

Children age two: 2 drops EO in 1 ounce (30 ml) of carrier oil

Newborn to children age two: 1 drop in 1 ounce (30 ml) of carrier oil

General Fluid Conversion Guide

1 ml = 20 drops EO
3.75 ml = 1 dram = ⅛ oz = 75 drops EO
5 ml = 1 tsp = 100 drops EO
15 ml = 3 tsp (1 tbsp) = ½ oz = 300 drops EO
30 ml = 2 tbsp = 8 drams = 1 oz = 600 drops EO

Dilution Guide for Safe Skin Application

How much essential oil should you put into your carriers for safe skin application? Generally, effective blends for adults are made using a dilution ratio of 1, 2 or 3 percent of essential oil to the carrier. Perfume oils are higher dilutions of 5–10 percent.

1% Dilution (5–6 drops per ounce [30-ml] carrier): Use for children under twelve, seniors over sixty-five, pregnant women and people with long-term illnesses or immune system disorders. A 1 percent dilution is a good place to start with individuals who are generally sensitive to aromas, chemicals or other environmental pollutants.

2% Dilution (10–12 drops per ounce [30-ml] carrier): Use for general health and skincare, natural perfumes, bath products and your everyday blends.

3% Dilution (15–18 drops per ounce [30-ml] carrier): Use for specific application blends and acute health conditions (i.e., treating a cold or flu, pain relief and sports blends).

5% Dilution (28–30 drops per ounce [30-ml] carrier): Use for sports massage blends, natural perfumes and short-term treatment for specific, acute health conditions.

10% Dilution (58–60 drops per ounce [30-ml] carrier): Very expensive essential oils like rose, helichrysum and neroli are often made available in a 10 percent dilution of carrier oil. Essential oil blends for natural perfumes and specific applications may sometimes also be found in 10 percent dilutions.

Medical Terms: Primary Actions and Effects

Adaptogens/Regulators: substances that promote beneficial adaptation to change; refers to the pharmacological concept whereby administration results in stabilization of physiological processes and promotion of homeostasis or balance

Analgesic: pain reliever

Antidepressant: alleviates or prevents depression, lifts mood, counters melancholia

Anti-inflammatory: reduces inflammation resulting from injury or infection

Anti-infectious/Antimicrobial: kills microorganisms or inhibits their growth

Anti-parasitic: inhibits and destroys growth of parasites

Antispasmodic: calms nervous and muscular spasms; for pain and indigestion

Carminative/Stomachic: settles digestive system, relieves intestinal gas

Cicatrizant: wound healing; promotes formation of scar tissue

Digestive/Stomachic: aids and promotes appetite and assists digestion of food

Expectorant/Mucolytic: promotes removal of mucus from respiratory system

Fungicidal: prevents and destroys fungal infection

Insect Repellant/Insecticide: repels and destroys insects

Rubefacient: increases local blood circulation causing analgesic effect

Sedative: promotes calming and tranquilizing effect and induces sleep

Stimulant: raises levels of physiological or nervous activity in the body; good for convalescence and physical fatigue

Urinary Tract Antiseptic: inhibits growth of microorganisms in the urinary tract

Psycho-emotional Aromatherapy Chart (Super Oils)

Action	Problem	EO Solution
Regulator or Adaptogen (either stimulant or sedative)	Manic/depressive, extreme mood swings, depressive anxiety, hormone imbalance	bergamot, geranium, rose, ylang ylang III, sandalwood, cedarwood, blue yarrow, helichrysum, frankincense, palmarosa
Motivating	Lethargy, boredom, issues of low self-worth, immune depression	grapefruit, rosemary, peppermint, lemongrass, eucalyptus, thyme
Sedative	Fear, stress, worry, insomnia, irritability, anxiety, anger issues	chamomile, sandalwood, ylang ylang III, red mandarin, melissa, neroli, spikenard, vetiver
Stimulant	Mental fatigue, poor memory, poor concentration, inability to focus	lemon, peppermint, cinnamon, rosemary
Uplifting (mood enhancer)	Loss of inspiration, lack of direction, aimless, purposeless	grapefruit, ylang ylang, tangerine, black spruce, peppermint, lemon
Relaxant	Stressed, uptight, control issues	clary sage, geranium, sandalwood, ylang ylang, sweet marjoram, palmarosa, lavender, frankincense
Euphoric	Depression, lack of self-confidence, moody	neroli, ylang ylang, grapefruit, clary sage, spikenard
Aphrodisiac	Shyness, isolation, loneliness, frigidity, emotional coldness, withdrawal, impotence, loneliness	sandalwood, cinnamon, ginger, clary sage, rose, patchouli

Symptoms Guide: Super Oils to Use

Adaptogen/Regulator: bergamot, geranium, ylang ylang III, rose, frankincense, sandalwood

Allergies: blue tansy, hyssop, ammi visnaga, chamomile, lemongrass, spikenard

Anxiety/Fear/Worry: bergamot, vetiver, ylang ylang, rose, neroli, melissa, geranium, clary sage, chamomile, red mandarin, black spruce, black pepper

Circulation: rosemary, cinnamon, ginger, peppermint, cypress, black pepper, black spruce

Congestion/Cough: eucalyptus, lemon, cinnamon, ginger, rosemary, hyssop

Cramps/Spasms: peppermint, black pepper, sweet marjoram

Depression: bergamot, sandalwood, geranium, rose, neroli, melissa, frankincense, ylang ylang, grapefruit, black spruce, sweet orange

Detoxification: juniper berry, lemon, rosemary

Digestive: ginger, peppermint

Fungal Infection: palmarosa, thyme, oregano, tea tree, grapefruit

Hormone Balance: geranium, rose, bergamot, clary sage

Infection: palmarosa, eucalyptus, clove, cinnamon, thyme, oregano, ravensara, tea tree, ledum

Inflammation/Burns: chamomile, helichrysum, lavender, blue tansy, blue yarrow

Injury/Wound Healing: helichrysum, rose, chamomile, sweet marjoram, rosemary

Insect Repellant: palmarosa, rose, geranium, patchouli, peppermint, cedarwood, lemongrass

Pain Relief: chamomile, peppermint, sweet marjoram, black pepper, ginger, black spruce

Parasites: cinnamon, clove bud

Respiratory: eucalyptus, hyssop, ledum, ammi visnaga, frankincense, blue tansy

Sedative: spikenard, vetiver, ylang ylang III, chamomile, red mandarin, lavender, clary sage

Skincare/Burns: geranium, carrot seed, lavender, chamomile, rose, ylang ylang, galbanum, frankincense, myrrh, sandalwood, patchouli, cypress

Stimulant: rosemary, ginger, lemon, peppermint, black pepper

Urinary Tract Infection: juniper berry, lemon, rosemary

Weight Control: grapefruit, lemon

Further Reading, Resources and References

The Practice of Aromatherapy: A Classic Compendium of Plant Medicines and Their Healing Properties, by Jean Valnet, MD, and Robert B. Tisserand

Aromatherapy Workbook, by Marcel Lavabre

The Secret Teachings of Plants: The Intelligence of the Heart in the Direct Perception of Nature, by Stephen Harrod Buhner

Clinical Aromatherapy: Essential Oils in Practice, by Jane Buckle

The Art of Aromatherapy: The Healing and Beautifying Properties of the Essential Oils of Flowers and Herbs, by Robert B. Tisserand

The Aromatherapy Practitioner Reference Manual (2 Volumes), by Sylla Sheppard-Hanger

The Blossoming Heart: Aromatherapy for Healing and Transformation, by Robbi Zeck, ND

The Complete Book of Essential Oils & Aromatherapy, by Valerie Ann Worwood

Aromatherapy for Healing the Spirit: Restoring Emotional and Mental Balance with Essential Oils, by Gabriel Mojay

Animal Aromatherapy Practitioner Certification Course[SM], by Kelly Holland Azzaro

The Magic of Ayurveda Aromatherapy: Discover the Magic & Rare & Unique Ayurveda Aromatherapy Oils in Harmony with Universal Healing Success, by Farida S. Irani

The Chemistry of Essential Oils, by David G. Williams

Aromatherapy: The Complete Guide to Plant and Flower Essences for Health and Beauty, by Daniele Ryman

Complete Aromatherapy Handbook: Essential Oils for Radiant Health, by Susanne Fischer-Rizzi

Aromatherapy for Health Professionals, 4th edition, by Len and Shirley Price

Aromatherapy Workbook: A Complete Guide to Understanding and Using Essential Oils, by Shirley Price

Medical Aromatherapy: Healing with Essential Oils, by Kurt Schnaubelt

International Fragrance Association, http://ifrafragrance.org

Essential Oils Safety: A Guide for Health Care Professionals, 2nd edition, by Robert B. Tisserand and Rodney Young

Acknowledgments

For my son, Ezra, my inspiration, who never gave up on me!

To my agent, Marilyn Allen, who, like an angel, found me and guided me through the publishing process.

Big thank-you to my editor, Liz Seise, my publisher, Will Kiester, and the Page Street team for their invaluable assistance in birthing a truly great book!

About the Author

KG is an earth-loving aromatherapist, metaphysical coach and holistic health educator of more than 35 years. She is passionate about helping others become the person they most want to be, by living a full life.

Born and raised in Wilmington, North Carolina, KG knew from a very young age she wanted to help people feel better. She realized early on it was the way people were thinking that caused most, if not all, of their problems. KG became passionate about changing the way people think about their life situations. After college, and with nothing more than a desire to help people overcome their challenges, she began pursuing her dream.

After discovering the work of Carl Jung and Rudolph Steiner, KG traveled to the Findhorn community in Scotland and became even more immersed in transformational healing. After being introduced to essential oils, she realized that she had found what she had been looking for her whole life. One sniff of pure plant essences can instantly shift a person's thinking and mental attitude.

KG is proud to have created a socially conscious online presence that positively touches hundreds of thousands of lives around the world. Her online aromatherapy training and metaphysical coaching programs help people, like you, live true to themselves, free to take meaningful action and create a life they love. She lives in Ashland, Oregon.

Index